Bukk G. Carleton, Charles Deady, William Francis Honan

A manual of genito-urinary and venereal diseases

Bukk G. Carleton, Charles Deady, William Francis Honan
A manual of genito-urinary and venereal diseases
ISBN/EAN: 9783337733438

Printed in Europe, USA, Canada, Australia, Japan

Cover: Foto ©ninafisch / pixelio.de

More available books at **www.hansebooks.com**

Genito-Urinary and Venereal Diseases,

—BY—

BUKK G. CARLETON, M. D.

Prof. of Genito-Urinary Diseases Metropolitan Post-Graduate School of Medicine of New York City, Visiting Physician to Metropolitan Hospital Dep. Pub. Char. and Corr. of New York City, Late Visiting Physician to Ward's Island Hospital, Late Pathologist and Interne Ward's Island Hospital, Late Adjunct Prof. and Demonstrator of Anatomy New York Homœopathic Medical College,

—WITH—

Venereal Diseases of the Eye,

By CHARLES DEADY, M. D.

Member of Board of Governing Surgeons New York Ophthalmic Hospital, Prof. of Ophthalmology and Otology College of New York Ophthalmic Hospital, Prof. of Ophthalmology Metropolitan Post-Graduate School of Medicine, Editor of the Journal of Ophthalmology, Otology and Laryngology,

—AND—

Vesical Calculus and External Urethrotomy.

By WM. FRANCIS HONAN, M. D.

Adjunct Prof. of Genito-Urinary Diseases Metropolitan Post-Graduate School of Medicine, Member of Auxiliary Board of Visiting Physicians to Metropolitan Hospital, Demonstrator of Anatomy New York Homœopathic Medical College, Late House Surgeon Brooklyn Homœopathic Hospital.

NEW YORK.
BOERICKE, RUNYON & ERNESTY.
1895.

PREFACE.

IT has been many years since a concise treatise on Genito-Urinary and Venereal Diseases, convenient for ready reference, has been offered for public consideration. The fact that many changes in the treatment have become necessary from a better understanding of the diseases themselves, the rapid advance in Antiseptic and Aseptic Surgery, and a better general knowledge of Bacteriology and its relations to cause and effect pointing the way in many cases to their more rational treatment, to say nothing of the new remedies and operations advocated in the past few years, are sufficient reasons in our judgment, for the presentation of this book.

General literature has been consulted in the preparation of these pages and proper consideration given to the treatment recommended. The scope and size of the book have precluded the mention of the details of many operations, some being given only in outline.

The question of dose has been left almost entirely to the individual prescriber. It has been the Author's desire to give only a short resumé of the diseases in question and their latest and most satisfactory treatment.

By the kindness of the publishers cuts of instruments have been inserted, thus obviating the necessity for their description.

The Author is greatly indebted to Dr. Chas. Deady for the complete chapters on Venereal Diseases of the Eye, as well as to Dr. Wm. Francis Honan for the papers on Stone in the Bladder and External Urethrotomy.

Extra space has been given to the consideration of Venereal

PREFACE.

Diseases of the Eye, as many eyes are ruined which 'could have been saved had the proper treatment been instituted early in the disease.

Many thanks are due to Dr. R. du Jardin for his able assistance in preparing the manuscript for the press.

With the knowledge of its many shortcomings this volume is submitted to the profession with the hope that it may prove a useful "vade mecum."

173 West 47th Street, New York City,
   March 1st, 1895.

CONTENTS.

CHAPTER I.

Diseases of the Prepuce and Glans Penis—Balano-Posthitis—Herpes Progenitalis—Vegetations—Preputial Calculi—Varices of the Prepuce—Epithelioma—Phimosis—Circumcision—Inflammatory Phimosis—Treatment.

CHAPTER II.

Special Therapy for the Prepuce and Glans Penis.

CHAPTER III.

Diseases of the Urethra—Gonorrhœa—Chordee—Peri-urethral Folliculitis—Bastard Gonorrhœa—Urethritis—Gleet—Stricture: Spasmodic, Organic, Traumatic, Linear, Annular, Irregular—Treatment—Sounds—Divulsion—Internal Urethrotomy—External Urethrotomy: Gouley's, Wheelhause's and Cock's Operation—Electrolysis: Newman's Method—False Passages—Retention of Urine from Stricture of Small Calibre—Urinary Extravasation—Treatment.

CHAPTER IV.

Gonorrhœa in the Female—Treatment.

CHAPTER V.

Special Therapy for Urethral and Gonorrhœal Discharges.

CHAPTER VI.

Urethral and Urinary Fever—Treatment.

CHAPTER VII.

Gonorrhœal Rheumatism—Treatment.

CHAPTER VIII.

Gonorrhœal Affections of the Eye—Gonorrhœal Conjunctivitis—Gonorrhœal Iritis: Plastic Form, Serous Form—Treatment.

CHAPTER IX.

Diseases of Cowper's and the Prostate Glands—Cowperitis—Prostatitis: Acute, Chronic or Follicular—Hypertrophy of the Prostate—Treatment.

CONTENTS.

CHAPTER X.

Diseases of the Bladder—Cystitis: Acute, Chronic—Irritability or Neuralgia of the Neck of the Bladder—Incontinence of Urine—Retention—Strangury—Treatment.

CHAPTER XI.

Stone in the Bladder—Vesical Calculus—General Consideration—Clinical History — Non-Operative Treatment of Stone—Operations: Perineal, Lateral, Median and Supra-pubic Lithotomy, Litholapaxy—Stone in the Female Bladder.—Treatment.

CHAPTER XII.

Pyelitis: Acute, Chronic, Calculous, Tubercular—Gravel—Renal Calculi—Renal Colic—Treatment.

CHAPTER XIII.

Special Therapy for the Prostate, Bladder, Ureters and Pelvis of the Kidney.

CHAPTER XIV.

Diseases of the Scrotum and Testes—Pediculosis Pubis—Erythematous Intertrigo—Prurigo—Elephantiasis Scroti—Testicles: Hypertrophy, Atrophy—Cryptorchid —Monorchid — Hydrocele: Acute, Chronic, Congenital, Encysted—Hydrocele of the Cord—Diffuse Hydrocele of the Cord — Encysted Hydrocele of the Cord — Hæmatocele—Encysted Hæmatocele of the Cord—Epididymitis—Orchitis: Acute, Chronic, Specific—Hernia Testis—Cysts of the Testis—Cancer of Testicle—Tubercular Testis: True, False—Castration — Neuralgia of the Testicle—Varicocele—Treatment.

CHAPTER XV.

Special Therapy for Diseases of the Scrotum, Testicle and Cord.

CHAPTER XVI.

Functional Diseases of the Genital Organs—Impotence: True, False—Sterility: Aspermatism, Azoospermism, Misemission — Masturbation—Satyriasis— Nymphomania—Priapism— Pollutions— Spermatorrhœa—Treatment.

CHAPTER XVII.

Special Therapy for Functional Disorders of the Genital Organs

CHAPTER XVIII.

Chancroid: Gangrenous, Phagedænic, Follicular, Diphtheritic—Treatment: Preventive, Abortive, Symptomatic.

CONTENTS.

CHAPTER XIX.

Bubo: Simple, Virulent, Specific—Treatment.

CHAPTER XX.

Special Therapy for Bubo.

CHAPTER XXI.

Syphilis: General History—Primary Stage, Clinical History—Twenty-three Diagnostic Points as considered with Chancroid—Treatment.

CHAPTER XXII.

Secondary Stage—Syphilitic Fever—The Syphilides: Roseola, Papular, Pustular—General Superficial Syphilides: Acne, Superficial Ecthyma, Pigmentary, Vesicular, Bulbous, Tubercular, General, Circular Groups, Squamous, Treatment.

CHAPTER XXIII.

Alopecia—Clinical History—Treatment.

CHAPTER XXIV.

Onychia—Paronychia—Treatment.

CHAPTER XXV.

Lesions of the Mucous Membranes in Secondary Syphilis—Mucous Patches—Scaly Patches.

CHAPTER XXVI.

Syphilitic Lesions of the Eye—Conjunctiva, Cornea and Sclera—Conjunctival Chancre—Mucous Patches—Conjunctival Gummata—Gummy Scleritis—Keratitis Parenchymatosa: Vascular Form, Non-Vascular Form—Kerato-malacia—Treatment.

CHAPTER XXVII.

Uveal Tract—Iritis: Plastic Form, Papular Form, Gummy Form—Cyclitis — Irido-Choroiditis — Choroiditis — Choroido-retinitis — Opacities Vitreous Humor—Treatment.

CHAPTER XXVIII.

Retina and Optic Nerve—Retinal Irritation—Diffuse Retinitis—Central Recurrent Retinitis — Papillitis — Papillo-retinitis — Retrobulbar Neuritis—Atrophy Optic Nerve—Amaurosis—Hemianopsia.

CHAPTER XXIX.

Lids, Lachrymal Apparatus, Orbit—Motor Nerves—Chancre of Lids:

CONTENTS.

Papular, Pustular, Ulceration, Gummy Infiltration — Gummy Tarsitis—Dacryocystitis—Lachrymal Stricture—Pre-Lachrymal Abscess—Dacryoadenitis—Orbital Periostitis: Acute, Chronic—Paralysis Third Nerve—Sixth Nerve—Fourth Nerve—Treatment.

CHAPTER XXX.

Tertiary Syphilis: Cutaneous Diseases—Ecthyma—Rupia—Pustules—Ulcerations: Superficial, Deep—Gummata of the Skin—Treatment.

CHAPTER XXXI.

Lesions of the Mucous Membranes—Mucous Patches—Circumscribed Ulcerations—Treatment.

CHAPTER XXXII.

Lesions of the Tongue, Larynx and Lungs—Gummata of the Tongue—Larynx: Erythema, Superficial Ulceration, Gummatous Lesions—Lungs: White Hepatization, Fibrinous Interstitial Pneumonia, Gummata—Treatment.

CHAPTER XXXIII.

Lesions of the Alimentary Tract—Liver: Diffuse Parenchymatous Hyperplasia, Gummata—Syphilis of the Spleen—Kidneys: Congestive Nephritis, Specific Nephritis—Treatment.

CHAPTER XXXIV.

Lesions of the Bones, Cartilage, Muscles and Tendons—Treatment.

CHAPTER XXXV.

Lesions of the Nervous System in Syphilis—Cephalalgia—Hemiplegia—Aphasia—Chorea—Epilepsy—Paraplegia—Insanity—Coma—Treatment.

CHAPTER XXXVI.

Marriage and Pregnancy of Syphlitics.

CHAPTER XXXVII.

Hereditary Syphilis—Treatment.

CHAPTER XXXVIII.

General Treatment of Syphilis.

CHAPTER XXXIX.

Special Therapy for Syphilis.

Illustrations.

Ricord's Circumcision Forceps	Fig. 1
Otis' Endoscope	" 2
Otis' Perfected Urethroscope	" 3
Kiefer's Two-Way Urethral Nozzle	" 4
Universal Soft-Red Rubber Syringe	" 5
Otis' Urethrometer	" 6
Bulbous Bougie	" 7
Keyes–Ultzman's Deep Urethral Syringe	" 8
Meatotomy Knife	" 9
Civiale's Meatotome	" 10
Weisse Sounds	" 11
Conical Steel Sounds	" 12
French Cylindrical Urethral Sounds	" 13
Thompson's Divulsor	" 14
Otis' Urethrotome	" 15
Bates' Urethral Hæmostat	" 16
Teale's Gorget	" 17
Gouley's Tunneled Catheter	" 18
Symes' Staff	" 19
Newman's Electrolysis Sounds	" 20
Banks' Whalebone Bougie	" 21
Winternitz's Psychrophor	" 22
Thompson's Stone Searcher	" 23
Silver Catheter with Long Curve	" 24
Soft Elastic Rubber Catheter	" 25
Mercier's Catheter, One Elbow	" 26
Mercier's Catheter, Two Elbows	" 27
English Catheter	" 28
Nitze Electric Cystoscope	" 29
Marcy's Double Current Catheter	" 30
Grooved Lithotomy Staff	" 31
Lithotomy Scalpel	" 32
Probe-pointed Lithotomy Knife	" 33
Curved Lithotomy Forceps	" 34
Bigelow's Lithotrite	" 35
Bigelow's Evacuator	" 36
Keyes' Varicocele Needle	" 37
Fusing Lamp	" 38

GENITO-URINARY DISEASES.

CHAPTER I.

DISEASES OF THE PREPUCE AND GLANS PENIS.

BALANO-POSTHITIS.—Balanitis is an inflammation of the glans penis, and posthitis an inflammation of the mucous lining of the prepuce. As one condition cannot continue for any length of time without developing the other they are considered together. The disease in itself, is not contagious, unless of venereal origin.

Etiology.—Predisposing causes: A long and tight prepuce, unclean habits and a gouty or strumous diathesis. The exciting causes are traumatism, the abnormal accumulation of smegma from the glands of Tyson, contact with menstrual, leucorrhœal, lochial or gonorrhœal discharges; it occurs also as a result of herpes, vegetations, chancroid or chancre, etc.

The clinical history will vary from a slight itchy, uneasy feeling behind the corona of the glans, with some redness or slight abrasion of the parts, accompanied by a yellowish or greenish-yellow discharge, to a case in which the discharge is profuse, greenish, purulent and offensive, the membrane swollen and œdematous, of a dark bluish-red or mottled cast, with irregular erosions of the epithelium here and there, especially in the region of the corona. The disease begins at this point and works its way forward on both balano and preputial surfaces. As the urine passes over the parts there is burning and biting in proportion to the degree of inflammation. With this condition there may be associated an inflammatory phimosis.

Prognosis.—Where the condition of the parts allows of perfect cleanliness and antisepsis, recovery will be rapid; but when caused by other disorders, the duration will depend in a great measure upon the original cause.

Treatment.—Cleanliness is of the first importance, without it recovery cannot ensue; but as alkalies (soaps, etc.) irritate they should be avoided. The parts should be bathed every two to six hours with one of the following solutions: Carbolic acid, 1 to 400; Hydrarg. bi-chloride, 1 to 5000; a saturated solution of Boracic acid; Succus Calendula, or Ernesty's Aqueous Hydrastis, 10 drops to the ounce of hot water; then dry (without rubbing) with absorbent cotton, if the parts can be exposed; if this cannot be accomplished, inject into the balano-preputial cavity (using a broad-nozzled syringe) some one of the solutions best adapted by its cleansing and antiseptic properties. The inflamed surfaces are then dusted with Sub-nitrate of Bismuth, powdered Alum or Tannin, and separated by a layer of absorbent cotton. If phimosis is present, frequent and prolonged immersion of the affected parts in hot water, made slightly antiseptic, will be necessary.

The remedies most frequently indicated for this condition are Mercurius, Coccus cacti, Nitric acid, Lycopodium, Aconite or Cannabis sativa.

HERPES PROGENITALIS.—When herpes appear on the integument of the penis or scrotum they differ in no way from similar lesions on other parts of the body, but on the mucous membrane of the penis their course is somewhat different. They are recognized by the development of one or a cluster of vesicles on a reddened and inflamed base, accompanied by a slight burning and itching. On the mucous membrane the vesicles become softened by prolonged maceration and break down, leaving an irregular, superficial, ulcerated surface, with more or less balanitis or posthitis, and if not properly treated may cause phimosis, or proliferate into vegetations. If the herpes develop in the urethra a discharge is invariably present.

Etiology.—Excessive venery; a depraved condition of the system; unclean habits and prolonged nervous strain or great anxiety. The disease tends to recur at frequent intervals on the slightest provocation.

Treatment.—Cleanliness: after washing with a weak antiseptic solution and drying, as in balano-posthitis, the vesicles and abrasions should be dusted with Sub-nitrate of Bismuth and Zinc oleate, equal parts; Calomel, Aristol or Merc. sol. Hahn. 1x, as indicated.

Preventive Treatment: Cold douches to the lumbar region for thirty seconds, twice a week; extra cleanliness and the local application of a little alcohol on the first indication of their appearance frequently prevents their development.

Remedies: Rhus tox., Croton tig., Thuja, Mercurius, when given according to their indications, not only hasten recovery, but tend to prevent the recurrence of the disease.

VEGETATIONS.—Condylomata or warts are papillary epithelial outgrowths which are very vascular.

Etiology.—Uncleanliness, especially in those with a long, tight prepuce; moisture. They frequently result from balanitis, herpes and venereal lesions.

Clinical History.—They are located most frequently in the fossa behind the glans penis, but may appear on the glans itself, the prepuce, in the urethra, on the scrotum, around the anus, as well as on the labia of the pregnant female, in fact on any part of the external genitals. They may be broad and flat, arranged like a cock's comb or pedunculated, single or multiple, and bathed in a fetid, purulent discharge.

Treatment.—Immediate removal, as there are good reasons for believing that they have developed into or were the cause of malignant growths. The pedunculated variety should be removed with curved scissors and the base cauterized with Nitric or Carbolic acid. The broad growths should be first painted with a 5 or 10 per cent. solution of Cocaine, then Pyrozone 25 per cent., or Nitric acid applied. After the vegetations turn white the surplus can be absorbed with cotton or blotting paper; if pain continues the application of a drop of Carbolic acid will stop it, or they may be painted with a saturated solution of Salicylic acid and Collodion; the action of the latter is slow, but free from pain. The parts in the meantime should be kept dry by dusting with some antiseptic and astringent powder, as Sub-nitrate of Bismuth, Tannin, Aristol or Dermatol. If broad, flat and numerous, and especially if located on the scrotum, the best treatment is the application of Calomel and the use of moderate pressure, when they will soon disappear. In some cases cleanliness alone has cured. If any doubt exists about diagnosis remove a small portion and examine under the microscope before commencing treatment. Remedies: Thuja, Nitric acid and Staphisagria.

PREPUTIAL CALCULI.—Children with a long prepuce and congenital phimosis are liable to this disorder. They result from a deposit of the salts of the urine in or around the corona, forming a calculus varying in size from a millet seed to a small hen's egg. They may exist for years as a hard tumor under the prepuce without producing annoyance or discharge, but in time a purulent flow results from its presence. If the prepuce is long and tight, a differential diagnosis from gonorrhœa, when the history is questionable, is sometimes difficult without a microscopical examination. Sounding with the probe will very likely clear up the diagnosis, unless the stone has become enclosed by an adhesive balano-posthitis.

Treatment.—Removal of the calculi. Circumcision.

VARICES OF THE PREPUCE are easily recognized by the unusual size of the veins.

Treatment.—Removal by circumcision or electrolysis. Special remedies: Hamamelis, Lachesis.

EPITHELIOMA seldom occurs before the 40th year; it is most frequent between the 50th and 60th years.

Etiology is obscure, but it has been thought that intercourse with a female suffering from cancer has, in some cases, been the exciting cause.

Clinical History.—It commences as a small, flat, warty growth or ulcerated surface with an indurated base, generally on the glans, rarely on the prepuce, with a tendency to the formation of a dark crust or scab, which, on being removed, leaves a granular, ulcerated surface, exuding a fetid, ichorous fluid, with burning and lancinating pains in the diseased parts. In time the inguinal glands become swollen, indurated and painful. The ulceration rapidly advances, the edges are everted, and sinuses lead off into the surrounding tissue, which soon becomes involved and destroyed. When ulceration has commenced the diagnosis can easily be made, but in all suspicious cases it must be verified with the microscope.

Treatment.—Excision of the diseased parts to prevent the fearful ravages which are sure to follow.

Marked relief has sometimes resulted from the exhibition of Arsenicum, Conium, Thuja, etc.

PHIMOSIS is a narrowing of the preputial opening.

Etiology.—It may be congenital or acquired, acute or chronic. Male children are usually born with a condition of phimosis and an elongated prepuce, but if this can be retracted so as to expose the glans, unless retained smegma or adhesions of the balano-preputial surfaces cause unlooked for symptoms, there need be no anxiety about the case. The preputial opening enlarges rapidly as the child advances towards puberty, allowing the glans at this time to be readily exposed.

Clinical History.—When the preputial orifice is not as large as the urethra, which is indicated by the ballooning of the prepuce at each urination, an operation is indicated. If neglected, the mechanical irritation from overdistention and urine remaining in the balano-preputial cavity will in time set up a balano-posthitis. If the preputial opening becomes red and inflamed, causing the child to pull on the parts or retain the urine for a long time simply because it hurts him to urinate, circumcision or the stretching of the prepuce will be indicated. This treatment also applies to cases where the meatus becomes red and puffy, the lips everted and irritated, or when numerous reflex symptoms, such as convulsions, spinal disorders, enuresis, result from adherent prepuce or retained smegma.

In adults a tight prepuce may require operation to prevent the serious results that herpes, retained smegma, etc., may produce with a narrow preputial orifice. The phimosis may be congenital or acquired from cicatricial contraction, from old chancres, herpes, or indirectly from inflammation of the integument.

Treatment.—In childhood surgical interference is frequently indicated.

In some cases it is best to circumcise, but in the majority the stripping back and dilatation of the prepuce, under proper antiseptic precautions, will suffice. In childhood the preputial opening will admit of being stretched so that the foreskin can be retracted behind the glans.

Stripping the glans should be executed under perfect asepsis. In this operation grasp the penis between the thumb and forefinger of the left hand and with the right thumb and index finger push the prepuce back; if the preputial opening is narrow introduce the point of a small pair of dressing forceps and open carefully to a moderate degree only, then repeat the stripping until successful. If there are adhesions between the glans and the inner surface of the prepuce break them up with a flat probe, but always continue the stripping until the fossa back of the glans is completely exposed and the smegma removed. Wash the parts with an antiseptic solution and dress with a Boracic acid or Calendula salve, the foreskin being returned over the glans, otherwise the parts may swell rapidly and paraphimosis might result. The dressing must be repeated daily by the surgeon until the balano-preputial membranes are in a healthy condition. This leaves the foreskin in a natural condition as a protector of the numerous nervous filaments which have their terminal fibres in the glans penis.

Except in phimosis in the adult, and from cicatricial tissue and thickened growths, or from venereal requirements the stripping operation is the most satisfactory one for the relief of phimosis.

Circumcision.—Perfect asepsis. Chloroform may be used up to the eighth year, but afterwards Ether should be used as the anæsthetic, or the hypodermic injection of Cocaine at the seat of operation may be employed. A probe is first passed into the preputial opening and swept around to break up the adhesions; the integument is then marked with an aniline pencil about a quarter of an inch in front of the curve of the corona, the parts being in a state of repose. Do not cut behind this mark. Bring the foreskin forward, grasp the prepuce with the circumcision forceps (Fig. I) applied obliquely, care being taken not to include

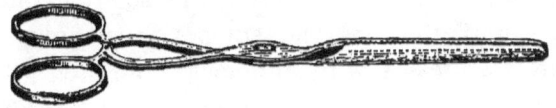

FIG. I.

in its grasp the preputial orifice. Remove the redundant tissue down to the aniline mark with curved flat scissors. After the removal of the external or skin layer of the prepuce slit down the mucous layer to the corona and trim to its edge, avoiding the frænum; break up the remaining adhesions and dress antiseptically. The use of hot water or torsion will usually control the bleeding, if not enclose the bleeding points in the horsehair sutures used to approximate the mucous and cutaneous surfaces. In very young children sutures are not necessary as the parts heal in about forty-eight hours. When sutures are used a large number may be reqnired; the tied ends should be cut about an inch long to prevent their sticking into the parts, which frequently swell and become œdematous during the first few days.

The first sutures should be placed one on either side of the frænum, and so situated as to tie in and control the frenal arteries, then the suture in the median raphé is tied tight, cutting into the skin. The others, as many as may be required, should be placed between and tied loosely. These sutures usually cut themselves out and are removed with the scab about the fifth day. If this should not occur they can be removed on the fifth to the seventh days. The operation is completed by placing a narrow strip of Iodoform gauze around the line of suture and held in place by Iodoform collodion, this is encircled by narrow strips of absorbent lint, which must be saturated frequently with a Hydrarg. bi-chloride solution 1 to 4000, or a solution of one teaspoonful of Carbolic acid and Glycerine, equal parts, to a pint of warm water, or a solution of Ernesty's Aqueous Hydrastis or Succus Calendula, a teaspoonful to the quart of warm water. The use of one of these solutions must be continued until the scab and stitches are removed, when the parts are dressed with a Boracic acid, Zinc oxide or Carbolic acid ointment. Sometimes œdema in a marked degree will occur after the operation, requiring the application of an ice-bag to reduce it.

The exhibition of Aconite, Arnica, Capsicum, Cannabis sat., Calcarea carb., Euphrasia, Mercurius, Rhus tox., Thuja, or Sulphur as indicated may in some cases make an operation unnecessary by rapidly relieving the distressing symptoms.

INFLAMMATORY PHIMOSIS is generally transitory, the prepuce being swollen, red and tumefied, with marked narrowing of the preputial opening. It is secondary to some other disease as balanitis, herpes, chancre, etc.

Treatment.—It is rapidly reduced by hot fomentations made slightly antiseptic, or Hamamelis solution, hot baths, rest in bed with the penis well carried up against the hypogastrium and retained there until the inflammation subsides, and the injection with a flat-nozzled syringe into the preputial cavity of some cooling or antiseptic solution, as Dilute Lead Water, etc. Should the inflammation continue and chancroid be suspected, or the circulation become interfered with, an operation is required.

PARAPHIMOSIS applies to that condition where a tight prepuce has been drawn over the glans and cannot be replaced. Such a condition if not relieved will in a short time lead to the most serious results.

Etiology.—It is usually caused by the inflammation accompanying herpes, chancre, balano-posthitis, etc.

Clinical History.—When once seen it will never be forgotten. The diagnosis is easy, the glans penis presents a congested, purple, or even gangrenous aspect; behind the corona rises a tense, œdematous, shining collar, back of this is a deep sulcus, most marked above, possibly ulcerated; in this band lies the stricture. Back of this sulcus rises another collar of œdematous tissue.

No time should be lost in relieving this condition, or it may result in gangrene and consequent loss of the parts. Where strangulation is moderate it will produce intense local pain and constitutional disturbances.

Treatment.—When the œdema is excessive small punctures may be made in the œdematous collar to reduce the œdema and thus facilitate replacement. If it is of recent origin anoint the parts with some antiseptic oil, then place thumbs upon the glans and with the first and second fingers of both hands grasp the penis behind the swelling on their respective sides and with the thumbs pressing the glans back and the fingers drawing the œdematous parts forward the paraphimosis can be reduced. If this treatment is not successful the glans may be wrapped with an elastic band and compressed so that it can be slipped *through* the constricted collar with the handle of an instrument. Should all manipulation fail the constricting band must be cut, but always remember that it is the *second* band that is to be cut; this can be done from within outwards with a flat bistoury.

When reduction is easily effected the parts are dressed with a solution of Hypericum, Opium and Lead-water, or a solution of Carbolic acid and Glycerine, equal parts, one teaspoonful to a pint of warm water. Arnica, Apis, Mercurius or Calendula as required internally.

CHAPTER II.

SPECIAL THERAPY FOR THE PREPUCE AND GLANS PENIS.

Acidum Nitricum.—Denuded spots with itching, throbbing and pressure on glans penis, also flesh-colored excrescences exuding an offensive moisture and bleeding on touch; superficial ulcers, looking clean but exuding an offensive matter; itching-tickling like the bite of small insects within the prepuce. Moisture on glans and prepuce. Itching vesicles on prepuce that open and become covered with thick matter. Swelling of penis. Phimosis without much redness, accompanied by ulcerating surfaces on prepuce and at the margin of the meatus urinarius. All erosions bleed easily. Sharp, stinging pains.

Acidum phosphoricum.—Oozing vesicles around the frænum. Crawling and itching in vesicles. Stitches in glans penis. Heat and sore pain in warty growths when walking and sitting. Erection in morning and feeling of weariness in the glans.

Aconitum.—Stitching, crawling and stinging pains in the glans and prepuce; prepuce swollen and inflamed; pinching pains in the glans on urinating; the patient is restless, anxious, with more or less fever.

Apis mel.—Inflammation and great œdema of penis, with sharp, stinging pains. Burning and stinging pains on urinating. Warty excrescences.

Arnica.—Inflammatory conditions from mechanical violence; stitches through the glans; itching of the parts. Erections after walking.

Arsenicum.—Painful swelling of penis with burning pains; itching in glans which is blue, red and cracked. Corrosive pain in penis; stitching and itching pains on the end of prepuce; inflamed, bleeding surfaces.

Belladonna.—Soft, painless pimples on the glans; prepuce retracted behind the glans, causing disagreeable feeling; itching and biting on fore part of glans; frequent erections; smarting on outer edge of prepuce after urinating.

Bryonia.—Glans covered with a red, itching rash.

Caladium.—Glans covered with red points; dryness of glans penis, with a desire to rub; prepuce swollen along its margin. Sore and painful, with biting on urinating, compelling rubbing. Sore, corrosive pain in prepuce.

Calcarea carb.—Cutting and burning on glans penis. Prepuce inflamed and red, with burning pain on touch and on urinating.

Cannabis sativa.—Moisture about the corona; glans red and covered with dark spots; penis is painful, as if excoriated or burnt, when walking; prepuce dark-red, with heat, swelling and inflammation; burning and corrosive pains in the glans penis with exudation; constant burning of the glans and prepuce; burning on urinating, with excoriation of the preputial opening.

Cantharis.—Inflammation, heat, swelling; pain and itching of glans penis. Gangrene. Red, hot and shining swelling of prepuce, with phimosis and discharge of purulent matter from beneath it; discharge of blood. Pruritus. Pain on urinating. Brown, cheesy accumulation behind the corona, in the morning.

Capsicum.—Constant pressure in the glans, with bruised sensation; aggravation morning and evening. Itching and stinging like the bite of insects.

Carbo veg.—Vesicles on the inner side of the prepuce, with itching and soreness.

Causticum.—Red spots or herpetic redness with oozing on glans and frænum. Vesicles under the prepuce becoming suppurating ulcers. Burning pains in penis; itching on inside of penis; at other times burning and biting. Increased secretion of smegma.

China.—Burning in glans and prepuce. Jerking pains between the glans and prepuce when walking. Itching of the glans in the evening. Sore sensation on the margin of the prepuce. Tearing pains in left side of prepuce and in left testicle.

Cinnabaris.—Red spots on glans penis as if pimples would form, with itching and burning of corona glandis relieved by rubbing, then aggravated with exudation of much pus of a nauseating, sweetish smell. Warts on the prepuce, bleeding from the slightest touch, with swelling and itching; soreness on urinating. Itching in the fossa behind the glans; jerking in penis; stitching pains in the glans.

Coccus cacti.—Pustule in the middle of penis. Throbbing in the glans. Heat and itching in the glans. Biting and stitches in the prepuce.

Colocynthis.—The prepuce is always drawn back and constricted behind the glans at night. Tearing and pricking in the glans.

Conium.—Inflammation of the prepuce. Sticking and

cutting pains in the prepuce. Tearing pains through the penis when not urinating. Itching of the prepuce and glans not relieved by rubbing.

Copaiva.—Excoriation of the glans and prepuce. Tickling and itching of the glans. Discharge profuse and milky with much burning and smarting.

Corrallium rub.—Red, flat ulcers on glans and prepuce with a yellowish discharge. The glans and under surface of the prepuce secrete a yellowish or greenish offensive matter with redness, swelling and sensitiveness of the organ to touch. Swelling of the prepuce with sore pain on the edge when it rubs against the clothes. Pain in the frænum as from needles. Ulcers bleed easily and exude an offensive moisture.

Croton tig.—Inflammation of the inner surface of the prepuce with irritation of the parts and some secretion. Burning in the glans on urinating. Redness of the glans. Vesicles on the penis. Herpetic eruption on the scrotum. Corrosive itching of the scrotum and glans. Moist offensive spots and desquamation of the epithelium of the glans.

Euphrasia.—Sticking pain on tip of glans. Voluptuous itching of glans when sitting, becoming painful after scratching. Voluptuous itching on the margin of the prepuce, and pressing pains after scratching. Slight watery discharge from the parts.

Gelsemium.—The glans and prepuce are swollen and congested with irregular red spots over the membrane.

Graphites.—Glans penis covered with thick mucus. Tension of parts aggravated by contact with the clothing when walking, with pinching, jerking and drawing pains. Vesicles on prepuce and other parts, with voluptuous itching. The prepuce swollen like a large water-blister without pain. Itching and moist eruption.

Hamamelis.—Itching, tingling and throbbing pains in the glans and prepuce. Enlargement of the veins of the penis, which is inflamed and painful.

Hepar sulph.—Itching and sticking pains in the glans penis and scrotum. Ulcers on prepuce with fetid discharge. Profuse, offensive discharge around the glans penis. Herpes of the prepuce very sensitive to touch. Vegetations discharging an offensive pus. Inguinal glands involved and suppurating.

Ignatia.—Excoriation on margin of prepuce with ulcerative pain and itching. Biting itching on inner side of prepuce and glans. Sore pain in frænum and glans as if excoriated.

Kreosotum.—Vegetations with profuse, foul-smelling pus, with much burning and smarting.

Lachesis.—Red pimples beneath margin of the corona glandis. Red spots on glans with jerking pains and profuse discharge. Gangrenous condition.

Lycopodium.—Redness and inflammation of prepuce with great itching of its inner surface and of the frænum. Yellow exudation behind the corona glandis, with dark red, soft elevations, and biting, itching and tearing in this region. Much smegma behind the glans.

Mercurius.—The most important and most frequently indicated remedy in balano-posthitis. The prepuce swollen as if distended with water. Swelling and inflammation of both glans and prepuce, with more or less discharge. Fine, red eruptions. Cracks and chaps, with burning biting itching and voluptuous pain. Red vesicles on the glans, which become ulcers. Profuse muco-purulent discharge and involvement of the inguinal glands. Herpes of the prepuce; the abraded surfaces itch and sting if pressed or bathed.

Mezereum.—Obstinate cases with profuse discharge from the glans with excoriation in the fossa behind; tearing, burning and lancing pains. Itching in the prepuce, especially after urinating. Swelling and inflammation of prepuce. Itching and burning vesicles.

Natrum carb.—Itching, burning and stinging in the

prepuce, glans and frænum. Prepuce inflamed, glans swollen, sore and painful. Smegma behind glans.

Natrum mur.—Offensive secretion. The prepuce is retracted from the glans, causing a dry sensation; aggravated by walking and contact of the clothing. Itching of the corona glandis with moisture. Itching with crawling and prickling pains in the glans, which is red at the tip with red elevations. Offensive-smelling smegma. Jerking, throbbing, rhythmical pains in glans and frænum; greenish discharge.

Nux vomica.—In gouty individuals; sore pain, burning, biting and itching in glans, especially after urinating. Corrosive pain morning and evening. Prepuce retracted behind the glans penis, with soreness of its margin, with biting and itching on the inner surface of the prepuce. Increased smegma behind the glans; abrasion of the membrane when the prepuce is retracted. All symptoms are worse towards evening.

Petroleum.—Tearing, itching pains in the glans, with red spots or a reddish eruption; sticking pains on urinating. Herpes.

Pulsatilla.—Tickling, itching, biting and crawling pains, sometimes agreeable, referred to the glans penis towards morning or in the evening and when sitting, sometimes accompanied by a discharge of prostatic fluid. Constrictive pain behind the glans, with pressing pain after urinating. Itching beneath the prepuce.

Rhus tox.—Redness and swelling of the glans penis, with burning and biting in the urethra after urinating. Swelling of the prepuce, dark red on its inner surface, with sticking and itching pains and moist eruption; the prepuce looks and feels as if scalded, the vesicles exuding a transparent fluid. Vesicles on the glans and on prepuce, with intense itching, soreness and smarting.

Sarsaparilla.—Herpes on prepuce. Secretions have an intolerable odor. The glans is red and inflamed. Tearing pains from the glans to the root of penis after urinating. Pimples which burn and itch and become moist after scratching.

Sepia.—Red spots on glans, which are almost raw, coming and going on the glans and inner side of the prepuce. Tickling on touch. Discharge of a sour, salty-smelling fluid, with great itching and soreness. Sometimes a pale eruption on glans, with or without itching.

Staphisagria.—Soft excrescences around the glans, with an offensive discharge. Moisture around the corona beneath the prepuce. Moist growth behind the corona, with itching from rubbing of the shirt. Sticking pains in right side of the glans, when standing.

Sulphur.—Redness of the glans and inner surface of the prepuce, with soreness, burning and smarting. Pimples and pustules on the glans and desquamation. Fetid smegma, causing burning, smarting and itching, or discharge of a viscid mucus, which bites and burns. The parts are sometimes ice-cold. Redness of the glans; the prepuce is stiff and hard, with shooting pains. Prepuce red, swollen, with burning pain.

Thuja.—Condylomata, with sticking pain. Dirty, flat ulcers on the glans, surrounded by redness and sticky discharge, with burning pain. The glans is covered with a foul-smelling, yellowish-green secretion. Eroded spots, surrounded by red margins; sensation as of granular elevations. The sebaceous glands of prepuce are inflamed. Depressed vesicles, with stinging pains when urinating. Meatus red and puffy. Excoriated feeling near the frænum. Itching on glans and prepuce when walking, alternating with pain in anus. Burning in tip and excoriated feeling in the glans when urinating. Sensitiveness to touch. Reddish excrescences behind the glans penis. Red spots with inflammation on the inner surface of the prepuce. Red, eroded spots, exuding a thin, yellow, foul-smelling discharge. The prepuce is swollen, with red, condylomata-like growths on the surface; on the inner surface a red, moist tetter, depressed in the middle, painful to the touch, with burning and itching in the glans and prepuce; aggravation in afternoon. Dirty looking ulcers and growths.

CHAPTER III.

DISEASES OF THE URETHRA.

Any inflammation of the urethral mucous membrane is a urethritis, but all urethral inflammations do not necessarily constitute gonorrhœal infection, as they may be caused by mechanical and chemical agencies, individual idiosyncrasies, vegetations, herpes, chancroid or chancre within and upon the urethral mucous membrane; cases resulting from cold and exposure have also been recorded; therefore no urethral discharge should be pronounced true gonorrhœa without the best of proof or a bacteriological examination, and even then there are cases in which the gonococcus so found does not necessarily indicate a new specific infection. In cases of urethritis of a gonorrhœal character the gonococcus of Neisser will always be found, and if absent, the disease is not contagious, and therefore not of gonorrhœal origin.

GONORRHŒA.—This is the most frequent disease of the urethra the physician is called upon to treat, and the most contagious of all the venereal diseases.

Etiology.—It has but one mode of origin, that is the contact of a discharge containing the gonococcus of Neisser with a mucous membrane. Abrasion of the tissue is not necessary to make infection sure. No other cause is required.

Clinical History.—In from one to twenty-one days after coitus with a person suffering from gonorrhœa, but usually in about four days afterwards, there is noticed a slight tickling, crawling or itching at the meatus urinarius; the lips may be glued together or there may be present the smallest amount of a bluish, milky, sticky discharge. During the first five days, which period may be called the advancing stage, the symptoms rapidly multiply, the discharge becomes profuse and assumes a yellowish, purulent or greenish-yellow color, the green color depending upon the admixture of a little blood from the rupture of the over-distended vessels, and which may sometimes be so marked as to give a distinct bloody character to the discharge. As the disease travels backwards it may involve the glands of Cowper, the prostate, neck of the bladder or testes.

The urethra becomes sore, aching, and tender to touch, micturition becomes both frequent and painful, and is accompanied by burning and smarting; retention of urine rarely occurs unless the patient continues to drink and carouse while the discharge is progressing, or where the disease has been engrafted on an old and tight stricture. The meatus becomes œdematous, red, swollen and puffy, and may be accompanied by more or less balano-posthitis and even phimosis. If the inflammation is severe it will extend to the corpus spongiosum producing congestion and inflammation with an exudation into the elastic tissue of which it is composed. This exudation may occur at any point between the fossa navicularis and the triangular ligament; it interferes with the elasticity of the tissue forming the corpus spongiosum, hence when the corpora cavernosa become swollen and erection of the penis takes place, the corpus spongiosum being unable to expand and elongate is drawn tight like a bow string, giving rise to the exquisitely painful condition known as chordee.

The chordee should never be broken, as was formerly advised; this forcible extension, while giving immediate relief to the pain, causes hæmorrhage, and later, traumatic stricture; but if the penis be bent gently in the direction of its concavity the pain will cease and the parts soon become flaccid. The lymphatics on the dorsum and side of the penis are frequently involved, feeling like cords under the skin. Should the lymphatics of one side or the top of the organ be most affected, the corpus spongiosum remaining unaffected, erection may produce a deflection (chordee) to either side or upwards. The inguinal glands are occasionally involved, becoming swollen and painfully sensitive; sometimes suppuration occurs.

If the disease extends backwards the testes may eventually be attacked, causing an epididymitis. Examination of the urethra by the Otis endoscope (Fig. 2) or his perfected urethroscope (Fig. 3) reveals a congested, inflamed, red and swollen mucous membrane, with here and there spots of erosion of the epithelium, and the folli-

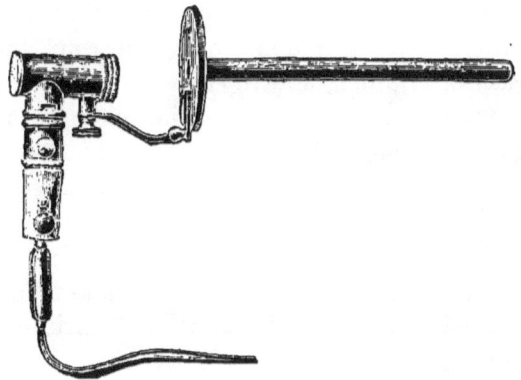

FIG. 3.

cles of Morgagni discharging a muco-purulent fluid.

This stage is liable to last from one to two weeks and is followed by the stationary stage, of variable duration, in which there is no special change; this, in turn, is followed by the third or receding stage, recognized by the gradual disappearance of the inflammatory

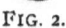

FIG. 2.

condition from the canal, but frequently leaving at the bulb or at the fossa navicularis, where the general inflammation usually is most severe, irregular patches of inflamed membrane. This may soon subside and the parts ultimately return to a healthy condition. Sometimes at the opening of the sub-mucous ducts there will appear granulations which may develop into vegetations. The ducts themselves may become plugged, causing peri-urethral folliculitis or abscesses, which can be felt beneath the skin along the course of the urethra as rounded masses, varying in size from a millet seed to a small pea. They are movable but held by a cord which is the obliterated duct of the gland.

The infiltrated submucous tissue may gradually thicken and contract, causing stricture; this anatomical change may prevent the symptoms entirely disappearing, and there will remain a frequent desire to urinate, with a slight discharge in the morning, or a mere drop at the meatus, without other symptoms being present; in other words, a gleet or chronic gonorrhœa.

Treatment.—This condition calls for remedies which will not only cure the urethritis, but must also possess a germicidal action, as Copaiva, Eucalyptus, Terebinth, Thuja, Ichthyol, Erigeron, Mercurius and Kreosotum, while Aconite, Gelsemium, Cannabis sat., Cantharis, etc., will be required for the simple inflammation.

BASTARD GONORRHŒA.—Etiology.—When the urethra has been damaged by former disease a purulent discharge may be caused by venereal excesses associated with overeating and drinking, even when the woman is in every way free from disease. In the gouty and strumous it may occur without sexual indulgence, simply from excesses at the table, chilling of the extremities, overfatigue from any cause whatever, or prolonged ungratified sexual excitement.

Clinical History.—Within a few hours after an indiscretion there appears at the meatus a slight discharge of muco-pus, some uneasiness, with or without increased frequency of micturition, and possibly accompanied by a slight burning and smarting, with much mental anxiety from previous experience.

Treatment.—Under the appropriate remedy and hygiene the symptoms rapidly disappear and in a few days an apparent cure results; they should, however, be warned of the probable condition of their urethra, and after a proper time, when the discharge has abated, a thorough examination of the urethral canal should be instituted and treatment directed to the cure of the original lesion so as to prevent future trouble.

URETHRITIS.—Etiology.—Traumatism of sufficient duration and intensity [as excessive and prolonged coitus], contact with various discharges, as leucorrhœal, lochial, menstrual, etc., ulceration of the uterus, acid urine, passage of urinary calculi, foreign bodies in and the passage of instruments through the urethra, colds, etc. Persons of a lymphatic temperament are especially liable to this disorder. This condition is usually associated with some individuality or excess.

Clinical History.—In all cases great care must be taken and conclusions must not be jumped at in diagnosing the various urethral inflammations. When in doubt look for the gonococci with the microscope; they appear like little black dots, arranged in pairs, fours, sixes or lines, and may be seen within the pus cells, differing from the urethrococcus. These also resemble black dots, but appear *outside* of the pus cells and are not arranged regularly.

The microscopal examination of a suspected discharge is made as follows: Spread a drop of the fluid over a clean, thin glass cover, hold this by means of a pair of forceps in a current of hot air over an alcohol lamp until dry, then apply a drop of the alcoholic solution of methyl-violet and allow it to flow over the dried discharge; the surplus may be removed by turning the glass with its edge resting on a piece of blotting paper, which will absorb it; then dry as before; then allow a small stream of distilled water to flow over the discharge, so as to wash off the dye. Repeat the drying process and the technique is completed by applying to the specimen a drop of Canada balsam dissolved in Benzol; this soon spreads over the cover, which should be placed on the slide ready for examination.

The symptoms commence as in gonorrhœa, only they are confined to the first inch of the urethra and rarely assume the severity of specific urethritis, and usually subside in a few days. Sometimes, however, the inflammation becomes exceedingly violent.

Treatment.—Cleanliness and the exhibition of the indicated remedy usually cure the case completely in a few days.

General consideration of the treatment of urethral discharges requires remedial, symptomatic, chemical, aseptic, antiseptic, mechanical and hygienic measures varying with the cause and course of the disease.

There are many remedies which rapidly cure simple urethritis and the gleety exacerbations known as bastard gonorrhœa, with or without antiseptic or astringent measures, as Aconite, Gelsemium, Cantharis, Cannabis sativa, Capsicum, Nux vomica, Sulphur, Thuja, etc. When the disease is caused by the gonococcus of Neisser, we must have remedies which not only cure the urethritis but also by their presence cause the destruction of the gonococcus. Many remedies have this two-fold action, $i.\ e.$, Copaiva, Sandal-wood, Cubebs, Ichthyol, Mercurius, Kreosotum, Erigeron, Thuja, and Nitric acid.

If the urethritis is non-specific no better remedies than Aconite, Gelsemium, etc., can be used during the advancing stage, but when specific Mercurius cor., Copaiva, Ichthyol, etc., will be more frequently indicated.

When the gonococci are present in the urethral discharge and the remedy prescribed does not have this two-fold action, the treatment, unless supplemented by various antiseptic or astringent injections, will be far from satisfactory. However, if they do combine this double action and are administered in the proper dose, the results are frequently brilliant.

If granulations, abrasions or strictures result with gleety discharges, etc., local and mechanical treatment will be indicated, such as the passage of sounds, local applications, etc., to the inflamed membrane, though many cases of gleet are perfectly amenable to the properly indicated remedy. The rapid and complete recovery depends largely upon the hygienic care and antisepsis which these cases receive.

The classical treatment requires rest in bed until the discharge ceases. Some cases so treated have delighted the patient and physician by their unusually rapid recovery. Few can do this, but they can refrain from over-exertion, etc. A suspensory bandage should be worn when walking or standing, and they should sit or recline as much as possible. The companionship of women must be avoided.

The mind should not be allowed to dwell on sexual subjects. All urethral discharges contra-indicate the use of wines, malted liquors, and in fact any beverage containing alcohol. Water in large quantities should be advised, preferably the Poland and Clysmic.

Diet should be light and non-stimulating, the more milk, especially skimmed-milk, they drink the more rapid, as a rule, is the recovery.

If the foreskin is large it may be utilized to retain pieces of lint cut an inch square and placed over the glans. These can be moved and reapplied as required. This dressing absorbs the discharge and prevents soiling of the linen. Where the foreskin has been removed a penis bag can be worn connected with the suspensory bandage, or a few pieces of toilet paper can be wrapped around the penis, twisted at the end, and thrown away as soon as soiled.

The acidity of the urine greatly irritates the inflamed membrane in its passage outward, consequently an alkali, like Bicarbonate of Soda (10 grains three or four times daily), should be administered, or Vichy may be drank frequently.

The tendency to chordee may be combatted by Camphor (5 drops of the tincture in water every four hours), Bromide of Camphor (2 grains every three hours), Clematis, Gelsemium, or Lupulin; Aconite or Belladonna if feverish and restless. Traditional medicine recommends large doses of Bromide of Potassium, Monobromate of Camphor; also

℞ Antipyrin, ... gr. xv.
    Potassii Bromidum, ... gr. xlv.
M.
In one or divided dose at bed-time.

This painful condition may be greatly relieved by holding the penis in ice-water, or placing by its side a piece of cold steel, or ice, etc., or washing it in cold water four to six times daily for five minutes at a time. Inflammatory phimosis will require Aconite, Apis or Belladonna. Irritation of the neck of the bladder yields kindly to Cantharis, Aconite, Belladonna, Berberis, Prunus spinosa, Camphor, or Sabal serrul.; if not, the following may be used:

℞ Ext. Hyoscyamus,
    Ext. Cannabis Ind., ... āā, gr. viii.
    Sacch. Alb., ... gr. xlviii.
M.
Ft. Chart. No. xx.
Sig. A powder as required.

As a rule injections should not be advised during the advancing stage of urethral catarrh when the remedies are acting satisfactorily; yet any weak antiseptic solution— Bichloride of Mercury 1 to 40,000 to 1 to 20,000—as a douche, injected by Kiefer's two-way tube (Fig. 4) attached

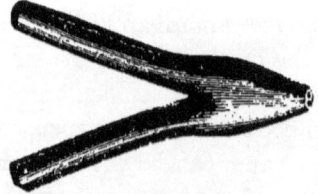

FIG. 4.

to a fountain syringe, one or two quarts each time, have been reported to act satisfactorily.

During the secondary stage of a severe acute gonorrhœal urethritis the remedies most frequently indicated are Copaiva,* Sandal-wood,† Cubeba, Kreosotum, Argentum nitricum, Ichthyol, etc. During this stage the remedies internally administered may be supplemented by injections of the same remedy when it has a germicidal action and is of vegetable origin, in the general strength of ten drops of the infusion or oil to the ounce of hot distilled water. Not more than one or two drachms should be used at each seance. Hydrastis is frequently used in this manner, but more often Bichloride of Mercury 1 to 30,000 to 1 to 20,000; Nitrate of Silver, 1 to 4,000 to 1 to 2,000; or Ammonium Sulpho-ichthyolate, 1 to 100, as urethral douches.

The reason for the kindly action of the mild antiseptics at this stage is due to the fact that early in the case the specific virus is located superficially in the epithelium, while later it often gains entrance into the deeper layers and is protected by its position from germicidal injections. Experience teaches that many cases are rapidly cured by the Bichloride douche. Some after using it from six to twelve days apparently recover, but relapse when the treatment is discontinued, while in others the discharge does not stop but becomes thin, serous and colorless, even when the treatment is continued. These cases require astringents to complete the cure.

Care must be taken in using these douches not to overdistend the urethra or to send the injection beyond the first few inches of the pendulous portion of the urethra;

---

*The first decimal dilution and the tincture act kindly, but better results are generally obtained by the administration of two or three of the following pills after meals and at bed-time:

℞ Cera Alba, ... ℈iv.
    Balsam Copaivæ, ... ℈viii.
    Pulv. Magnesia, ... q. s.
Ft. mas. pil. Div. in pil. āā, gr. v.

† Acts best in 10-drop doses of the oil in capsules, taken after meals.

injections should not, under any circumstances, be thrown into the canal with force.

The universal soft red rubber syringe, with a single flow (Fig. 5) can also be used.

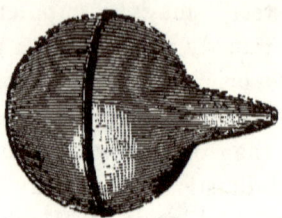

FIG. 5.

Hydrogen peroxide (in the strength of 3 to 5 volumes), or Pyrozone (one per cent. solution) can be used to advantage. In the declining stage astringents sometimes are called for, then a three-drachm hard rubber syringe, having a blunt, soft rubber nozzle, which expands rapidly, should be used. Never use a syringe with a long nozzle, as it irritates the urethra in the region of the fossa navicularis and may be the cause of stricture.

To properly use urethral injections the patient should sit on the edge of a chair with a roll of toweling behind the scrotum, pressing up against the bulbo-membranous junction, to prevent the injection from travelling backward and causing unpleasant complications. Grasp the penis between the thumb and index finger of the left hand, slightly retract and open wide the meatus; then, holding the syringe with the thumb and second finger of the right hand (the first finger being in the ring of the piston), the nozzle is tightly approximated to the meatus and the requisite amount of the solution slowly injected. Increased pressure is then applied by the thumb and forefinger at the meatus, permitting the syringe to be removed and the injection retained for a minute or two and then allowed to flow into a receptacle. This technique prevents soiling the linen, etc.

Never use an injection which produces an uncomfortable feeling or pain, the first few times, unless well acquainted with the individual urethra, dilute it with two or three times its volume of water until you are satisfied as to the strength you should use. Injections may be used from one to three or four times daily, always after urinating, taking advantage of the fact that the germicide or astringent is applied at a time when the canal has been well washed by the passage of urine.

Among the solutions which have given the most satisfaction as urethral injections are the following:

℞ Zinc. Sulph., ... gr. 1 to 2
Aqueous Ext. Hydrastis (Ernesty's), . . ℨ 1 to 2
Aqua, ... ℨii.
M.

℞ Zinc. Sulpho-carbolate, ... gr. 2 to 5
Aqua Rosae, ... ℨi.
M.

℞ Zinc. Permangan., ... gr. ss. to 1
Aqua, ... ℨi.
M.

Or a pure sedative, as:

℞ Acid. Boracic., ... ℨii.
Ext. Opii Aqueous, ... gr. xv.
Liq. Plumb. Subacet. Dil., ... ℨvi.
M.

For cases which linger with a tendency toward granulations, and where the disease remains in the submucous follicles and ducts, then

℞ Bismuth Salicylat., ... ℨii.
Acid. Boracic., ... ℨiii.
Liq. Hydrogen Peroxid., ... ℨvi.
M.

will act kindly.

Many others are recommended, but those already mentioned have been found the most useful.

When a slight gleety discharge persists, brilliant results are frequently obtained by the administration of tincture of Sulphur (in five drop doses, three times daily), Mercurius cor. 3x, Nux vomica in gouty cases, or Pulsatilla, Hydrastis, Clematis, Capsicum, etc., as indicated.

When examination of the urethra with the Otis urethrometer (Fig. 6) or bulbous bougie (Fig. 7), gives evidence of

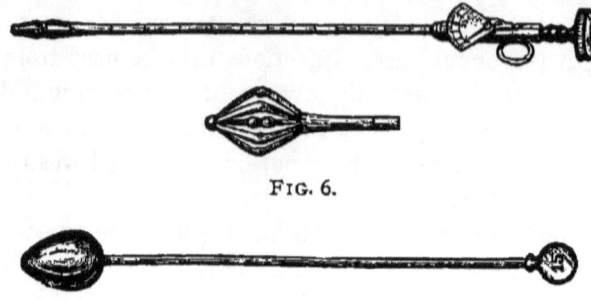

FIG. 6.

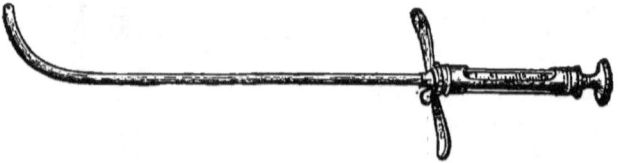

FIG. 7.

a small spot of granulation or urethral inflammation, the local application with Keyes-Ultzman's deep urethral syringe (Fig. 8) of one or two drops of solution Nitrate of

FIG. 8.

Silver, ¼ to 60 grains but usually from 4 to 10 grains to the ounce, will give the most satisfaction, applied every third day.

The best results are obtained by commencing with the weakest solution and increasing the strength as indicated, using an instrument devised by Prof. R. W. Taylor. About thirty drops of a solution of 1–2000 to 500 is taken into a one-ounce glass syringe with rubber trimmings, with nozzle drawn to a sharp point. A No. 8 French gum catheter is cut eight and a half inches in length and introduced (with the patient standing), to the indicated point, when the tip of the syringe is introduced into the catheter and the proper amount of the solution injected. The catheter is then removed and a piece of absorbent cotton, held by the foreskin or elastic band, is worn for a few hours to protect the linen from surplus dribbling.

If the granulations are large and numerous they may be successfully treated through the endoscope with Nitrate of Silver 4 to 40 grains to the ounce, applied by means of a pledget of cotton on an aluminium probe. These applications should not be made oftener than once in from 4 to 8 days.

In other cases the steel sound will be necessary to stimulate the parts and set up a healthy action in order to bring about the absorption of the newly formed tissue in and around the urethra.

During the receding and declining stages much will depend upon the building up of the general condition of the patient.

In many cases the discharge is prolonged by over treatment, and rapid recovery occurs on its discontinuance.

After treating a case of bastard gonorrhœa always locate the unhealthy portion of the urethra, which is usually found as a granular spot or a commencing stricture, possibly a stricture of large calibre left from an old urethritis, and which sometimes occur as a result of even the mildest cases. They must be given the proper care and attention.

There are cases when the indicated remedy will not act satisfactorily, where aseptic and antiseptic treatment are required, where urethral injections are objectionable from some particular reason, or it is desired to reinforce a urethral injection, then Salol is very beneficial, as it decomposes in the system into Carbolic and Salicylic acids, and as such is eliminated by the kidneys, and in its exit it comes in direct contact with all of the urethral mucous membrane. The same can be said of Sodium salicylate.

The abortive treatment of urethritis is generally believed to do more harm than good.

Under the proper treatment nearly all urethral discharges

that do not contain the gonococcus recover in a few days, or at most in 3 or 4 weeks; but those in which it is present will run a course of a few weeks, and occasionally, when occurring in a damaged urethra or where neglected, especially in the early stages, will persist for a long time to the discomfort of both the patient and physician.

The folliculitis which accompanies urethritis may require the administration of Capsicum or Sepia, but is usually relieved by the remedy covering the general condition. Should suppuration threaten or occur and is not dissipated by Hepar or Mercurius the abscess may break and discharge into the urethra or by adhesive inflammation attach itself to the skin and open externally. Silicea and Hekla lava may here be of benefit, or enucleate and dress the wound antiseptically. **Lymphangitis** can be cured by the indicated remedy, as Belladonna, Apis or Mercurius. **Adenitis** may require Aconite, Belladonna, Hepar sul., Mercurius, etc., with hot Calendula fomentations or the local application of Iodine, etc.; if suppuration supervenes open and dress antiseptically. **Cowperitis** will require Sabal serrul., Hepar sul., etc., with hot fomentations, hot poultices and rest in bed. If they do not relieve and resolution does not occur, an early incision before suppuration takes place should be made.

If the inflammation travels back and involves the neck of the bladder it produces a cystitis; when this occurs the gonorrhœal discharge ceases, returning when the bladder complication is relieved. This cystitis will require the administration of Cantharis, Belladonna, Camphor, Sabal serrul., Gelsemium, Aconite, etc. (See Diseases of the Bladder.)

STRICTURE.—This may be defined as an unnatural narrowing of the urethral canal. Three kinds are recognized—reflex or spasmodic, organic and traumatic.

SPASMODIC STRICTURE—Etiology.—It may be the result of natural, local or general conditions. The local being exemplified in the spasmodic condition complicating an organic stricture, of which we become cognizant when the sound is grasped as it passes through the contracted aperture. Sometimes a large sound can be passed through a stricture without difficulty, or if grasped by the spasmodic contraction firmly, easy pressure without force will cause relaxation and allow of instrumentation, while a small sound may be caught and held fast.

It may be reflex from hæmorrhoidal or other diseased conditions of the rectum or sacrum, dislocation of the hip, or a narrowed meatus. The general causes are: Chilling of the surface, irritation of the skin; even fright and anxiety will sometimes produce it.

One author of note claims that most deep strictures are spasmodic in character, caused by a narrowed meatus, and are speedily relieved by the proper meatotomy.

Clinical History.—Spasmodic strictures appear suddenly and immediately disappear on the removal of the cause. They always relax under complete anæsthesia. Cold, anxiety, etc., sometimes cause spasmodic stricture, resulting in retention of the urine. This condition appears suddenly. They are unable to urinate; in other words, to relax the compressor urethræ, or muscular coat of the membranous urethra.

Treatment.—Hot sitz baths and hot fomentations are indicated. If this condition is not relieved within a reasonable time a catheter must be passed. When this is not possible anæsthetize and use the catheter or aspirate to give the patient immediate relief, assuring him at the same time that the next urination will be normal.

Camphor or Gelsemium (5-drop doses of the tincture), Aconite or Cantharis 1x usually give us the happiest results, though Belladonna and Nux vomica or Prunus spinosa may also be called for. Traditional medicine advises Opium in one-grain doses every hour until natural urination occurs.

In all spasmodic strictures if you can find the cause and remove it, the stricture will immediately disappear.

ORGANIC STRICTURES.—These may be either congenital or acquired. The congenital are usually found at the meatus, while the acquired appear between the fossa navicularis and the bulb; in other words, in the first four inches of the urethra. They result from the contraction of newly-formed tissue in the corpus spongiosum.

Organic strictures may be linear, annular, or irregular in form.

The **Linear** are thin bands of tissue thrown across the canal, possibly in a semicircle or as a thin curtain with an opening in any part of it. This opening may be central, though not necessarily so.

The **Annular** are broad and flat, not over half an inch in width, encircling the canal.

The **Irregular** includes all other forms.

Strictures are also classified as of large and small calibre, the large being all those which allow of the passage of a No. 10 American or No. 15 French sound, while those of small calibre take sounds of a lesser size.

Most strictures are situated in front of the triangular ligament, occasionally they are found in the membranous, but never in the prostatic portion.

When strictures have existed for any length of time, they not only narrow the canal at their point of formation but ultimately lead to dilatation behind them. It is in this situation that a drop or more of urine lodges, to dribble away after micturition, the strictured condition preventing the onward impulse of blood through the corpus spongiosum that normally drives the urine forward in the urethra. The small quantity that usually remains behind the stricture undergoes decomposition; the changed urine attacking the mucous membrane causing granulations and an inflammatory condition. As the inflammation progresses and irritation still continues a mucoid secretion occurs, this is the source of the drop which is noticed at the meatus in the morning. There is also a slight smarting and an uneasy feeling as the urine passes over this spot.

The character of the urinary stream becomes changed, varying with the situation and size of the stricture, hence it may be small, forked or in driblets.

The strictured condition also interferes with the general circulation in the corpus spongiosum, giving the blue color to the glans penis so frequently noticed.

If the urine from one afflicted with stricture be placed in a glass vessel, strands or flakes will be seen to drop to the bottom of the receptacle, and the microscope will prove them to be little scabs or collections of pus corpuscles which have become detached from the granulating surface on or behind the constricted mass. The desire to urinate becomes more frequent, and this symptom is often the only one complained of when treatment is sought. Sometimes there is retention of urine, irritability of the bladder, neuralgic pains in the urethra and reflex neuroses in other parts, impotence, etc. Strictures of small calibre may, from their size and interference with the flow of urine, finally cause structural changes in the bladder, ureters, pelvis of the kidney and in the kidneys themselves.

The urethral canal must not be considered as a tube of equal diameter throughout its whole extent or that all narrowed points are strictures. It is found that it has three natural narrow spots, one at the meatus, one about an inch further back at the terminus of the fossa navicularis, and one about 3 or $3\frac{1}{2}$ inches from the meatus at the point where the canal passes through the triangular ligament. When it is over-distended other bands can be demonstrated with the Otis urethrometer, or with bulbous bougies, but these do not come within the scope of stricture unless there exists unusual narrowing; they are seen as rings standing out like thin fibrinous bands of a brilliant white color, and the mucous membrane bulged on either side when the canal has been inflated with air while using the Lister urethroscope.

The average meatus admits a No. 20 American sound, which should pass through all parts of the canal without difficulty; the size of the normal meatus being the best guide to that of the canal although the Otis scale is somewhat larger, which is as follows: Given a penis 3 inches in circumference in a state of repose the urethra should take a 30 French sound; if 3¼ inches, a 32 French; 3½ inches, a 34 French; 3¾ inches a 36 French, and when 4 inches or more in circumference a 40 French sound may be passed. Most authors consider this to be over-distension, yet in some cases it is required before recovery can occur.

Strictures of the meatus, when congenital, often exist without injurious effects, but sometimes on account of reflex symptoms or to facilitate other treatment their removal may become necessary. As dilatation is impossible a meatotomy must be performed. Often the meatus is narrowed by a little fold of tissue, leaving a sac just behind the meatus urinarius, a condition which is easily recognized by the use of a probe which catches in the fold along the floor or roof as the point is carried forward on the anterior part of the urethra, or a bulbous bougie will demonstrate its existence.

Meatotomy is performed with a blunt-pointed knife (Fig. 9) as follows: Grasp and pinch the glans between

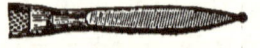

FIG. 9.

the thumb and first finger of the left hand; hold the knife in the right as you would a penholder, introduce it into the canal and cut through the stricture with an easy motion until all resisting tissue is divided. Civiale's meatotome (Fig. 10) may be used and gauged to the

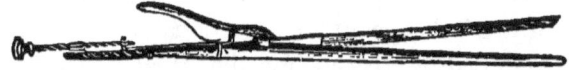

FIG. 10.

proper size by the Otis urethrometer. The incision is made on the floor of the meatus or on the roof should the pocket be above. The opening is generally made about two sizes larger than the normal canal, to compensate for retraction.

The operation is simple and not very painful. Cocaine, 4 per cent. solution, may be used as a local anæsthetic, but the wound does not heal as kindly after its use and bleeding will be more likely to occur. Hæmorrhage as a rule is not excessive; when profuse it may be controlled by the application of two pieces of veneer, about two by six inches, placed one on each side of the penis, and the pressure regulated by rubber bands or a piece of twine. After the bleeding has stopped they are removed and given to the patient to be used when required; the lips of the meatus may be pressed together and a drop of Collodion applied, the pressure to be continued until the Collodion dries. A Weisse sound (Fig. 11) should be passed daily for a week and also on the fourteenth day.

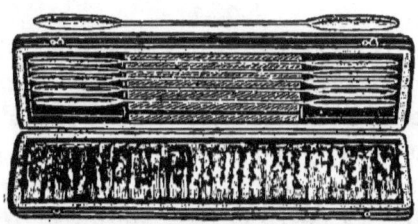

FIG. 11.

This treatment applies to all strictures situated within three-fourths of an inch of the meatus; these conditions are frequent, on account of the fossa navicularis being the seat of the severe localized inflammation in urethral diseases, and also the result of irritation arising from the longnozzled syringes formerly used in their original treatment.

Stricture of the pendulous portion of the urethra is easily diagnosed by passing into the canal a blunt-pointed sound the full size of the normal meatus. If it meets with an obstruction remove the sound and ascertain the size and length of the stricture with a bulbous bougie. (See Fig. 7.) Then the proper blunt sound is introduced through the stricture, which is felt as a band of firm, dense tissue encircling the instrument. The bulbous bougie may be used at first or the Otis urethrometer, especially if the meatus is contracted and when it is desired to ascertain at once the full diameter of the canal without performing a meatotomy.

A steel sound smaller than a No. 10 American or 15 French should not be used except by the most experienced operator. A blunt-pointed sound is used not only for diagnostic purposes, but also for relaxing spasmodic strictures. Conical-shaped sounds (Fig. 12.) are used for dilating,

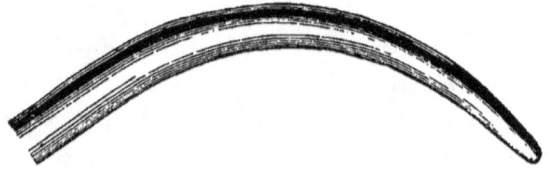

FIG. 12.

or, more properly speaking, for the absorption of strictures. They may be introduced in the following manner: The patient is placed in the dorsal position on a table, made as comfortable as possible and his mind diverted from himself. The surgeon standing on the patient's left holds the sound, which has been warmed and well lubricated, in his right hand, as he would a penholder, and grasps the glans and penis with the thumb and forefinger of the left hand; then, with the sound resting on or over the inguinal region, he introduces it, keeping the handle well down, allowing the penis to gradually swallow the instrument. When it has passed in about an inch beyond the curve the point of the sound will be at the opening in the triangular ligament; the handle is then carried to the median line over the abdomen and then brought down towards the feet, at the same time the scrotum is elevated by the disengaged fingers and the handle raised; then relaxing the hold on the scrotum, and possibly making a little pressure on the mons veneris, the sound sinks into the bladder as the handle is carried to a right angle with the body. Force must not be used, the sound should always enter by its own weight. Remove it with the same care and gentleness which should attend its introduction. If force is used more harm than good will result, preventing the relief which would otherwise have resulted from its scientific use.

Sounds should never be re-introduced until one or two days after the inflammation produced by their previous passage has subsided and absorption ceases, say about once a week.

In all strictures not admitting a No. 10 American steel sound the dilatation should be made with the French or English elastic sounds (Fig. 13); the progress is less rapid

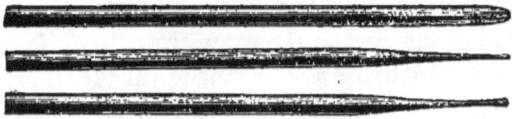

FIG. 13.

than with the steel sounds, but, on the other hand, they can be used every fifth day. At each instrumentation the sound first introduced should be two sizes smaller than the largest one used at the previous sitting, and then two, three or four introduced, one after the other, as judgment may dictate. To avoid urethral fever give five drops of Aconite 1x after instrumentation, especially to those who have not had sounds passed before.

Urethral fever may be the result of shock, but it occurs frequently when kidney trouble is present, hence the advisability of always examining the urine before passing the sounds, and to give Aconite for a few days before instru-

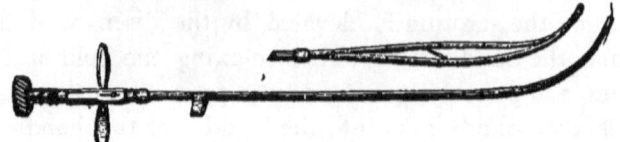

FIG. 14.

mentation in order to prevent shock.

Strictures of the pendulous portion of the urethra can be cured by the use of the sounds, and in many cases the symptoms removed by internal medication. Treatment by dilatation is slow, but it does not keep the patient from business, though in some cases, from want of time, when a rapid cure is desired or urethral fever follows instrumentation, divulsion with a Thompson divulsor (Fig. 14) may be indicated. This, however, has been largely superseded by the Otis urethrotome (Fig. 15), a dilator which dilates and cuts at the same time.

Internal urethrotomy is made on the roof of the canal, the cut being about two sizes larger than the measurements indicated by the urethrometer as the normal canal, the increased depth allowing for cicatricial contraction.

Do not make a second cut at the same place in the canal at one operation, but if necessary wait and do it later, as a second incision greatly increases the danger of urethral fever, etc. The operation is not very painful, and can be made without Ether. Hæmorrhage is sometimes profuse, but it can be controlled by compression or by the introduction

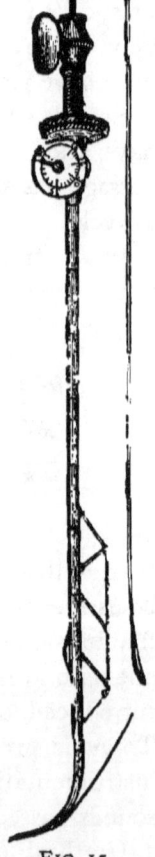

FIG. 15.

of Dr. Bates's urethral hæmostat (Fig. 16), which consists of a thin rubber tube arranged around a small catheter; it has an inlet and an outlet, through which ice-water can circulate freely, or it can be filled with air or water and the hæmorrhage stopped by its pressure; at the same time the urine can be withdrawn by unscrewing the cap of the catheter. When this instrument is not procurable the hæmorrhage can be controlled by the injection

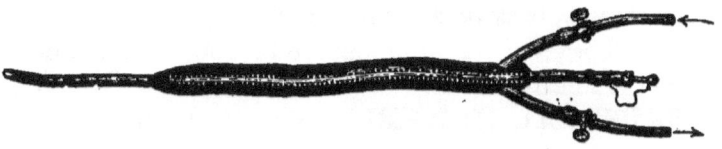

FIG. 16

of a drachm of the Solution Sub-sulphate of Iron, which is retained in the canal for a minute by pressure of the thumb and finger. When the pressure is removed a little watery fluid will escape from the meatus, but the canal will be effectually plugged by a solid clot. The only objection to this treatment is that suppuration is likely to follow and cause many unpleasant symptoms. The day following the operation and every second day for a week a full sized sound must be passed, after which time, in most cases, all symptoms will have disappeared.

In some cases the irregularities in the canal persist, and the weekly introduction of the proper sized conical steel sound for months will be necessary to complete the cure.

To use the Otis Dilating Urethrotome first locate the posterior border of the stricture with a bulbous bougie or the Otis Urethrometer. Introduce the urethrotome ¾ of an inch beyond its posterior border, as when the instrument opens the lower flange tends to draw the instrument forward. If this precaution is not taken the thickest and the most important part of the strictured band might escape division. Open the instrument to the desired size as indicated by the dial, exposing the knife in the groove, then drawing it forward through the stricture about half an inch beyond the distance indicated by the bulbous bougie, disengage the knife and withdraw the instrument, thus completing the operation.

In the membranous portion of the urethra dilate all strictures of large calibre unless resilient, and if possible those of small size; when this cannot be done and there is retention of urine or extravasation from rupture of the dilated canal, back of a small stricture, external urethrotomy will be required. Internal urethrotomy in this region is never indicated.

EXTERNAL URETHROTOMY.—If the stricture will admit of the passage of an instrument, it will require the simplest operation, which is generally spoken of as urethrotomy with a guide. The patient is anæsthetized, brought to the edge of the table and placed in the lithotomy position, with the hips well elevated. The perinæal and anal regions are shaved, and together with the thighs and buttocks scrubbed with soap and water, then douched with a Bichloride of Mercury solution 1 to 5000. The parts adjacent to the field of operation are wrapped in towels saturated with the Bichloride solution. A grooved staff is introduced into the urethra and passed into the bladder until the shoulder of the instrument presses against the anterior margin of the stricture. The staff is then passed to an assistant and the left forefinger introduced into the rectum. An incision with a small scalpel is made exactly in the median line of the perinæum, the shoulder of the staff being the objective point. When that is reached the knife is allowed to run in the groove of the staff, prolonging the incision towards the neck of the bladder until the strictured mass is entirely divided. The precautions to be observed are that the knife should always be in the groove of the staff, and that the stricture be thoroughly divided. The knife is withdrawn and a narrow probe-pointed Teale's gorget (Fig. 17) is introduced into the wound, its point following the groove in the staff until the bladder is reached, then a catheter is introduced into the penis, and passing along the gorget is guided into the bladder and then secured with tapes. The advisability of the retained catheter or perinæal drainage by means of a rubber tube introduced into the bladder

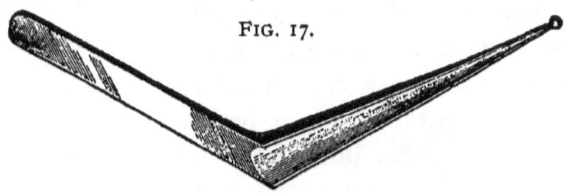

FIG. 17.

through the wound is a question which has provoked much discussion. Some surgeons, as Moullin and Gerster, do not favor either of the above procedures unless the urine is fetid. The weight of opinion, however, favors drainage with a tube or catheter, and also the washing out of the bladder frequently with a mild antiseptic solution. This combined with the internal administration of Boracic acid or Salol very effectually combats urethral fever. On the fifth day after the operation a steel sound is passed, to be repeated every three or four days until the wound heals. Its use should be persevered in for at least one year. If an instrument as large as the grooved staff cannot be made to pass the stricture, an attempt is made to pass a filiform bougie. This is done in accordance with the directions given in another section. If the attempt is successful the fact may be known by the ease with which the bougie can be moved. Over the filiform, as a guide, a grooved tunneled catheter (Fig. 18) is passed, and an attempt is made

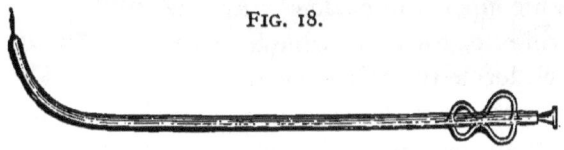

FIG. 18.

to cause it to pass the stricture. This can be accomplished in many cases. Great caution should be observed in this manœuvre, as the injudicious application of even a little force will sometimes do great damage to the urethra. Should the catheter be successfully introduced into the bladder the operation with the Symes' Staff (Fig. 19) differs in no way from the one previously described. If it will not pass, the tip of the instrument is pressed snugly against the stricture and an incision made in the median line of the perinæum until the bridged portion of the instrument is brought into view by opening the urethral canal. Long loops of silk are introduced into the lips of the wound so as to include the edges of the divided urethra. The black guide being located, the stricture is thoroughly divided with a narrow bistoury. The catheter is pushed into the bladder and the operation completed as before. When it is impossible to introduce a filiform bougie, the catheter may be passed as far as the stricture, the urethra opened, orifice of the stricture located, guide introduced, catheter threaded upon it and thus passed into the bladder. Finding the proximal orifice of the urethra in this way often requires much time and patience.

Pressure upon the bladder with the hand will often cause the urine to spurt, and thus locate the desired point.

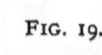

FIG. 19.

Supra-pubic cystotomy and retrograde catheterization have been recommended in some cases where an entrance

GENITO-URINARY DISEASES. 59

cannot be effected in the usual way on account of the failure to find the orifice of the canal. The above operation advised by Gouley, has largely superseded that of Wheelhause, which is similar, but requires a special staff, straight throughout and ending in a curved, rounded, button-like head. This is introduced into the urethra as far as the stricture and the canal opened up on the end of the staff about one-quarter of an inch anterior to the stricture.

Perinæal section, or Cock's operation, has always been considered a formidable operation, on account of the skillful technique required for its successful accomplishment. It consists in tapping the urethra at the apex of the prostate posterior to the obstruction, and, as it is performed without a guide other than the anatomical landmarks in that region, its difficulties are easily appreciated. It is well to have the patient retain his urine for some hours before the operation, as the consequent distention will cause

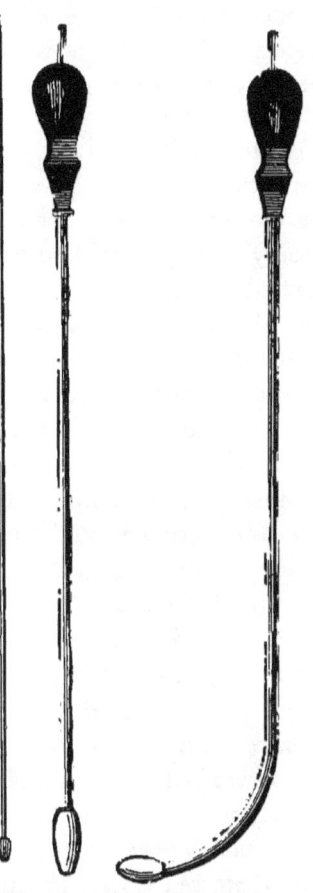

FIG. 20.

the posterior urethra to become more prominent. The lithotomy position is used as before, the patient lying as nearly straight as possible, so as to keep the part exactly in the median line. The operator's left forefinger is introduced into the rectum and the prostate located. An incision is made on the median line of the perinæum about one-half inch in front of the anus and carried steadily upwards towards the tip of the finger, then turned a trifle obliquely, when it will enter the urethra. Should the apex of the prostate be wounded it is a matter of no consequence. The knife is withdrawn, and the forefinger still being in the rectum a director is passed over it into the bladder.

In resilient stricture electrolysis succeeds in many cases and does away with the necessity for the more formidable operation of external urethrotomy. Newmans' electrolysis sound (Fig. 20) is selected and a galvanic current of not more than six milliamperes is used. The negative pole is connected with the sound and the positive with a large pad placed over the sacrum. The instrument should be lubricated with soap and water. While using the current easy pressure is made against the stricture. No force is allowed. The application should not be of more than ten minutes duration and never repeated oftener than once in five days. A second sound must never be introduced at the same sitting.

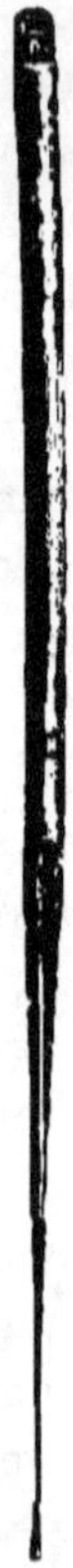

False passages are usually overcome and a sound may be passed by filling the canal and false passage with fine filiform bougies; Bank's (Fig. 21) serves all purposes best. By carefully and gradually applying the point of each the entrance to the bladder will usually be found and the stock can be pressed down, producing rapid dilatation, the fine filiform end bending upon itself in the bladder. After a few days a French or English elastic sound can be passed and dilatation continued.

FIG. 21.

The symptoms of stricture, even when instrumentation seems to be the only treatment required, will be greatly ameliorated by the exhibition of the proper remedy, *i. e.*

Nux vomica when the patient is irritable and there is digestive disturbance; Sulphur for general constitutional disturbances; Mercurius and Argentum nitricum when there is purulent discharge; Aconite and Cantharis for irritability of the stricture and neck of the bladder; also Capsicum, Clematis, Copaiva, Pulsatilla, Sandal-wood, Thuja, Silicea, Iodine, Kali hyd., Calcarea iod., etc.

Strictures of small calibre, when no indiscretions are indulged in, may go on without causing trouble, but chilling of the surface, exposure or over-indulgence of any kind may cause congestion of the parts and produce mechanical retention of the urine. This condition, if not relieved, may be followed by over-distention and atony of the bladder. If a catheter cannot be passed successfully relief must be obtained by the aspirator, the needle being introduced in the median line about half an inch above the symphysis. When the aspirator is used the bladder must not be entirely emptied, as violent shock might result if all the urine is removed. Administer a stimulant and apply an abdominal bandage for a short time after aspiration. Remedies: Gelsemium, Aconite, Belladonna, etc., in proper and repeated doses, frequently make the operation unnecessary.

When the stricture remains impassable external urethrotomy becomes imperative.

Urinary extravasation sometimes occurs from the sac back of the stricture and the urine burrows into the surrounding tissues; when small in amount it may be felt as a round circumscribed mass in the perinæum. When this occurs open and dress antiseptically.

CHAPTER IV.

GONORRHŒA IN THE FEMALE.

Etiology.—It has but one cause, the gonococcus of Neisser.

Clinical History.—The disease usually involves the vulva, vagina, cervix uteri and generally the urethra. If the disease is not checked it may extend to the body of the uterus, fallopian tubes, ovaries, etc., as we see in neglected or undiscovered cases, from which originate many of the disorders of the female pelvic organs.

The disease may make its appearance a few hours after coitus, but usually it has a period of incubation of about five days; if earlier, the symptoms are due to a great extent to excessive mechanical irritation of the parts.

At first there is a dryness and increased redness of the labiæ and vagina, with a feeling of heat and fullness, rapidly followed by a slight watery discharge, which soon becomes profuse, yellow, greenish, bloody and offensive. The labiæ and vagina become swollen, red and excoriated.

The disease frequently extends to the vulvo-vaginal glands, causing pain, swelling, and possibly abscess.

Micturition becomes frequent, and is associated with burning, smarting and tingling, as the urine passes over the external parts, whether the urethra is involved or not.

There is also heat, fullness and itching in the uterine, vaginal and perinæal regions, with marked tenesmus of the bladder and rectum.

The genital organs are frequently much swollen, especially when the vulvo-vaginal glands are involved; walking then becomes almost impossible. The disease may be accompanied by fever.

The history and the microscopical examination of the

discharge will make the differential diagnosis easy between the gonorrhœal and simple inflammatory vaginitis.

The duration of this disease is from three to five weeks, but if neglected it sometimes may last for years either at the cul-de-sac behind the neck of the uterus, in the cervix itself, or in the glands and ducts of Skene.

Treatment.—Rest in bed, with perfect cleanliness, antisepsis, and the indicated remedy, Aconite, Copaiva, Mercurius, Sandal-wood, Sepia, Sulphur, Thuja, Kreosote, etc.

Local antiseptic treatment is absolutely necessary in this disease. The indicated remedy will relieve the inflammation, but other means must be employed to eradicate the original and continuing cause; that is to say, the germs of Neisser. Alkalinity of the urine must be maintained to prevent and lessen the scalding as it passes over the inflamed labiæ.

Diet must be light and non-stimulating for the first two weeks.

The external parts must be kept clean by frequent bathing with Calendula, 1 to 100, or Borax, a teaspoonful to a quart of warm water, dried with absorbent cotton, and then dusted with Bismuth Sub-nitrate or Oleate of Zinc. Douches with two quarts of hot Bi-chloride of Mercury solution, 1 to 20,000, night and morning. Vaginal douches of Chlorate of Potash, two drams to two quarts of warm water, act very satisfactorily. Where the parts allow of the use of a speculum the daily introduction of a tampon, saturated with a mixture of Glycerine or Boro-glyceride with one-half dram of Bismuth Sub-nitrate gives good results. The Bismuth alone may be introduced into the vagina when instrumentation is painful, by means of a hollow capsule.

After the third week granulations remaining in the vagina or cul-de-sac should be dusted with powdered Alum or Tannic acid, and sometimes may require painting with a solution of Nitrate of Silver, 2 to 40 grains to the ounce.

Again, after apparent recovery every time after coitus her partner will in about five days develop a gonorrhœa. This is due to the persistence of the disease in the ducts and glands of Skene. By introducing the finger into the vagina and pressing upwards and drawing it forward along the course of the urethra a little drop of matter will be noticed exuding from these glands on either side of the urethra. This condition is easily overcome by injecting into each duct, with a hypodermic syringe with a blunt-pointed needle, a solution of Picric acid 1 to 1,000, or Nitrate of Silver, 4 to 40 grains to the ounce.

Condylomata are especially liable to develop in these cases, and require the same general treatment and remedies recommended for Vegetations, etc., on page 19.

CHAPTER V.

SPECIAL THERAPY FOR URETHRAL AND GONORRHŒAL DISCHARGES.

Acid Fluoric.—Gleet. Stricture. Gleety discharge during the night, leaving a yellowish stain on the linen. Frequent desire to urinate, with burning in the urethra.

Aconite.—Acute inflammation of the urethra, advancing stage. Burning when urinating with stitching pains in the meatus and fossa navicularis; fever, urine hot and burning. Great agony at the thought of urinating. Urine scanty and passed with difficulty. Burning at neck of bladder when not urinating. Crawling and stinging in the meatus and glans penis, which are inflamed, red and swollen. Copious, thick greenish discharge. Frequent painful erections at night; chordee. *Female.*—Heat, swelling and redness of external genital organs with frequent desire to urinate.

GENITO-URINARY DISEASES. 65

Agnus Castus.—Gleety conditions. Yellow discharge from the urethra. Disagreeable and uneasy feeling in back part of the urethra with frequent desire to urinate. Loss of sexual power and coldness of the parts.

Alumina.—Drawing and tearing pains in urethra in the morning. Burning after urinating. Frequent urination. *Female.*—Itching in pudendum. Burning in genitals, which are inflamed and corroded; patient is unable to walk. Amelioration from washing in cold water. Discharge profuse, and resembling the washings of meat. Lassitude and feeling as though the organs were prolapsed.

Argentum Nitricum.—Gonorrhœal urethritis. Frequently indicated in gonorrhœal and gleety discharges. Great burning in the urethra with frequent desire to urinate. Constricted, stitching feeling in the fore part of the urethra. Sensitiveness near the meatus. Inability to pass a projecting stream of urine, and a desire to pass a few drops immediately after urinating. Micturition difficult with burning and discharge of pus, shreds of epithelium and mucous membrane. Oozing of mucus from the meatus. Pain shooting from posterior part of urethra to anus and testes. Towards the end of urination sensation as if the urethra were knotted or closed. A feeling as if a drop of molten lead had passed along the urethra after urinating. Dragging, burning, stabbing pains along the urethra. Itching and tickling in the urethra. Discharge of blood and purulent matter. Chordee. Pain and swelling of the penis with slight fever. Enlargement of the testicles. Cutting pain in testes and cord. Stricture of the urethra.

Female.—Profuse, purulent and bloody discharge. Great soreness of the parts, which may ulcerate and bleed. Pruritus vulvæ.

Aurum.—Gleet. *Female.*—Profuse light-yellow discharge from the genitals. Burning and intolerable itching of the pudenda. Acrid leucorrhœa which excoriates the genitals. Induration of the inguinal glands.

Belladonna.—Micturition difficult. Tenesmus, the urine passed only in drops. Irritable strictures. *Female.*—Vagina hot and dry. Congestion and inflammation of the labiæ. Discharge of white mucus from the vagina, with violent stitches in the pubic region and inner parts; great pressure, as if the pelvic viscera would protrude through the vulva.

Calcarea Carb.—In females of lymphatic temperament. Milky discharge from the genitals with burning, biting and voluptuous itching of the parts, attended with pressure in vagina, which may be swollen, red and inflamed.

Camphor.—Strangury, violent, spasmodic and ineffectual efforts to urinate. Strangury not relieved by micturition. Retention of urine with a full bladder. Burning, biting and sticking in the urethra when urinating. Tenesmus of the neck of the bladder. Stream thin, as if the urethra was constricted. Acute urethritis with chordee.

Cannabis Sativa.—Advancing and stationary stages of urethritis. Difficult urination with constant urging and sensation as though the urine were tearing the tissues of the urethra. During urination burning, smarting and tingling in the urethra. Swelling of the prepuce (inflammatory phimosis) with dark redness of the glans. Penis feels sore and sensitive, the patient must walk with the legs separated. Burning during and after micturition. Discharge of watery mucus from the urethra. The urine spreads when voided. Meatus inflamed and painful to touch. Burning, biting pain extending backwards from the meatus on urinating. Pressure in fore part of urethra as if about to urinate when not urinating. Urine is scalding and burning, with frequent urging. Penis swollen, with sticking pains through the urethra. Swelling of the prostate. Urine bloody. Discharge may be moderate, or copious, white and yellow, with irritability of the bladder, or thin, watery, of a greenish-yellow color and offensive odor.

GENITO-URINARY DISEASES. 67

Female.—Cutting pain in the labiæ during urination. Urethra plugged with pus. Swelling of vagina.

Cantharis.—Urethritis. Strangury. Burning, cutting and scalding in the urethra during urination, with discharge of bloody mucus. Spasmodic pain at neck of bladder; tenesmus is almost unbearable, with constant ineffectual desire to urinate. Irritability of the neck of the bladder. Cutting pain before, during and after urination; the urine is scalding and passed drop by drop. Chordee. Discharge yellow and bloody. *Female.*—Burning heat of the external parts. Swelling of the vulva and vagina with itching, burning and a thick white discharge.

Capsicum.—Urethritis; yellow, purulent discharge from the urethra. Burning, biting, cutting pains in the urethra, between the acts of urination, most marked at the meatus. Tenesmus, strangury and almost ineffectual urging to urinate. Especially indicated in the fat and indolent with lax fibre.

Chamomilla.—*Female.*—Yellow, acrid, watery discharge, which smarts, burns and excoriates the parts.

Clematis.—Mucous discharge. Urinary flow irregular; has to wait some time before efforts to urinate are successful, with intense pain along the urethra, especially referred to the glans penis; commencing stricture.

Copavia.—Gonorrhœa. Inflammation of the urinary organs. Swelling and inflammation of the urethra, with pulsating pains through the penis. Constant, ineffectual desire to urinate; urine passed drop by drop, with burning and smarting in urethra and neck of the bladder. Itching, biting and burning in the urethra before and after urinating. Urine has the odor of violets. Meatus tumid, gaping and inflamed. Urination painful, with an acrid, milky discharge of corrosive character. Profuse, yellow, purulent discharge. Bloody urine, with frequent urination and chordee; violent erections at night. *Female.*—Itching of the vulva. Red spots on the vulva, with burning, milky leucorrhœa.

Cubeba.—Declining stage of urethritis and gonorrhœa. Dark reddish discharge from urethra; cutting and constriction after urination; inflammation of the penis. Urine has the odor of violets. Irritability of the urethra. Mucous discharge from the urethra. Absence of violent symptoms.

Digitalis.—Burning in the urethra, with purulent discharge, thick and bright yellow in color; frequent urging to urinate. Glans penis inflamed and covered with a thick, copious secretion of pus. Irritation of the neck of the bladder.

Erigeron.—Gleet. Gonorrhœa: receding stage. Burning, smarting on urinating; urine offensive. Drawing pains in the back, running down to the right testicle Chronic blennorrhœa, with irritability of the neck of the bladder.

Gelsemium.—Acute urethritis and dysuria from stricture.. Smarting and redness of the meatus ; burning at the meatus and along the urethra. Frequent urination, heat and little pain. Discharge moderate. Frequently used with good results in the early stage.

Ichthyol.—Has been given in cases of true gonorrhœa with brilliant results.

Kali Bich.—Ropy, stringy discharge from the urethra, in old cases of gleet.

Kreosotum.—Gonorrhœa and urethritis. Has been used in the male, but is most frequently indicated in the female. Great urging to urinate. Discharge bloody and very offensive, sanious, yellow, yellowish-white, foul, acrid, excoriating the labiæ, with itching and smarting. Corrosive itching within the vulva and on the labiæ. Burning, itching, and swelling of the labiæ.

Kali Hyd.—Urging to urinate, with pain. Thick, yellow-greenish discharge. Urethra irritable and sensitive.

Mercurius. — Gonorrhœa. Urethritis. Strangury. Urine passed with a feeble stream, with cutting pains. Lips of meatus red and inflamed. Swelling and burning. Glans penis dark red and hot, with burning, stinging, itching pains in the urethra. Discharge greenish, worse at night, thick and bloody. Muco-purulent matter mixed with the urine. Tenesmus. Painful erections. *Merc. Corr.* for more violent tenesmus, burning, and scalding; *Merc. Sol.* more burning between the urinary acts. *Female.*—Inflammation of the vulva, which is swollen, red, and hot. Pressing-down pain. Discharge of mucus tinged with blood. Copious discharge of watery mucus. Yellow leucorrhœa, with offensive odor.

Mezereum.—Discharge of watery mucus, increased by exercise. Itching of the prepuce. Heat, swelling, and titillation along the course of the urethra. Perinæum sore and tender to touch. Gleet.

Millefolium.—Swelling of the penis and testicle, with discharge of blood and watery slime.

Natrum Mur.—Clear, sometimes yellowish, discharge; cutting pain in urethra, after urination.

Nux Vomica.—When discharge has ceased there is complaint of irritation far back in the urethra referred to the neck of the bladder, with urging to urinate and to stool.

Pulsatilla.—Discharge of thick, milky mucus. Burning, stinging, and swelling of the labiæ.

Sandal-wood.—Receding stage of gonorrhœa. Stinging, smarting pain on passing urine. Redness and swelling of the meatus. Inflammatory phimosis. Discharge thick, yellow, or muco-purulent. Sub-acute attacks of urethral inflammations.

Sepia.—Gleet. Frequent urination, with burning and smarting in urethra, meatus, and neck of bladder. A remedy most frequently called for in chronic urethral discharges. Desire to urinate, with painful bearing down in the perinæum. Prostatitis. Stricture. *Female.*—Redness and itching of the labiæ and vagina, with discharge of yellow, greenish watery pus or foul smelling fluid.

Sulphur.—Gleet. Stricture. When other remedies well selected seem to do no good. Discharge thick and purulent, or thin and watery, with slight burning and smarting during urination. The urine is passed in a thin and divided stream. Itching in the middle of the urethra. Burning pains near the meatus, which may be red and inflamed. The walls of the urethra are thickened, when phimosis occurs, especially if there is inflammation and induration of the prepuce. *Female.*—Itching of the clitoris and burning of external parts, attended with a thin, burning discharge, especially in the morning.

Thuja.—Gleet. Burning in urethra. Crawling, burning, biting, piercing pains in urethra and meatus. Discharge thin and green between the acts of urination. Titillation, as though a drop of urine was passing along the urethra.

Tussilago Petasites.—Fixed pain in fossa navicularis. Profuse discharge. Inflammation of testes and eyes.

CHAPTER VI.

URETHRAL OR URINARY FEVER.

Etiology.—This disease has no known special anatomical lesion. It is recognized entirely by its clinical history. Some have attributed its origin to the absorption of decomposed urine, while others consider it purely a reflex or sympathetic affection. It is liable to occur during or after urethral or bladder instrumentation, especially in those suffering from some form of kidney disease, or in persons of an over-sensitive and highly nervous organization. Fatal cases have occurred in those who have had some nephritic disease.

Clinical History.—The gentle and careful introduction of a soft or a smooth conical steel sound has been followed by urethral fever, while a few days afterwards divulsion of the strictured urethra is often performed without unpleasant complications. Sometimes, even after a sound has been passed a number of times, a slight overdistention of the urethral canal by a larger instrument has resulted in urethral fever.

Urethral fever usually accompanies or follows within 24 hours of the first instrumentation; it does not necessarily appear with subsequent treatments. It occurs most frequently when the deeper portions of the urethra are operated upon, rarely from operations at the meatus. It has occurred when no damage of the urethra was apparent after death.

Well marked urinary fever from disease of the genitourinary tract has disappeared after the passage of sounds.

The severity of the symptoms varies greatly, most cases being slight in character. The disease is ushered in by a chill that does not occur until after urine has passed over the parts operated. There may be merely a slight coldness or a most pronounced chill followed by fever, perspiration and possibly delirium according to the severity of the chill. When the kidneys are healthy the symptoms pass off leaving the patient weak and depressed for a few hours or days, and complete recovery finally occurs. On the other hand, in those suffering from kidney disease there may be a marked chill, fever and perspiration, great prostration, anxiety, profuse vomiting and diarrhœa, suppression of the urine, uræmia and death in a few hours. Sometimes the chill and fever are mild, and yet symptoms of acute septicæmia or pyæmia rapidly follow, the autopsy often showing the presence of metastatic abscesses in the lungs, kidneys, liver, joints, etc.

Urethral instrumentation of the deeper parts may be attended or followed by urethral fever, hence the advisability of examining the urine before using instruments in order to eliminate as much as possible the dangers arising from their use. When instrumentation is imperative, place the patient in the best possible condition beforehand.

Treatment.—Preventive. If the urine is alkaline from decomposition, or gives evidence of nephritis, place the patient on a milk diet for a few days before instrumentation together with the administration of Salol, Salicylate or Benzoate of Sodium, to make the urine aseptic, and give Aconite 1x dilution or Gelsemium θ before and after passing the sound. Should the fever appear, Lachesis, China, Chin. arseniate, Rhus tox., Arsenicum, Phosphorus, Hepar sulph., Silicea, etc., as indicated.

CHAPTER VII.

GONORRHŒAL RHEUMATISM.

Etiology.—This disease is frequent in young men whose constitution is somewhat enfeebled either by excesses or overwork, or where there is an individual predisposition; females are rarely affected, though a condition somewhat similar is developed in women suffering from chronic endometritis, possibly of gonorrhœal origin. It has occurred in newborn infants following gonorrhœal ophthalmia.

It is supposed by many to be a slight form of pyæmia. Some believe it to be a reflex condition, and others look upon it as a systemic gonorrhœal infection.

Clinical History.—The disease appears in from six to eighteen days after the commencement of the gonorrhœal discharge, rarely after the second or third month. When it develops early it has no appreciable effect on the discharge, but later it has been noticed that the discharge increases somewhat for a day or two preceding the rheumatic outbreak. It develops in many forms, but has many characteristic individualities, attacking by preference the knee, ankle, sterno-clavicular articulation, and finally the joints of the foot and hand, in the latter case the tendons of the long muscles are liable to be involved as well as some of the bursæ. Those between the tendo-Achilles and the os-calcis are the most frequently attacked, becoming distended with a watery fluid, thus giving rise to the pain in the heel so often complained of by the gonorrhœal patient.

It frequently manifests itself as a mono-articular disease, usually selecting the knee-joint, which becomes distended with fluid accompanied by uneasiness and want of confidence in the joint, together with weakness and atrophy of the muscles of the thigh and leg; pain is rarely present. In the poly-articular form several joints are attacked one after the other, but those first involved continue to suffer during the attack and are the last to recover.

The joints are somewhat swollen and red with some fever, which is always less than in acute articular rheumatism, often lasting but a day or two. The tendons connected with the joints are generally involved and feel like thick bands; the conjunctiva become red and congested, the conjunctivitis frequently preceding the rheumatic symptoms. There is an entire lack of proportion between the local and constitutional symptoms. Perspiration, which is profuse in acute articular rheumatism, is characterized by its absence, and there is no change in the urine. The disease is tedious, frequently lasting for months, and recurrent attacks may lead to ankylosis. It does not move from joint to joint, and is rarely complicated with cardiac lesions. An attack occurring during a gonorrhœa predisposes to a return of the rheumatic symptoms with each subsequent urethritis or exacerbation.

The conditions are all relieved by rest, but the joints remain stiff long after the acute symptoms have disappeared. There is another variety characterized by a vague yet withal a very distressing and sharp pain in the joints without appreciable lesion.

Treatment.—Diet moderate, heathful and invigorating, avoiding anything that will increase the urethral trouble. The joints should be covered with absorbent cotton or flannel, and the parts must be given perfect rest until every vestige of inflammation disappears. The stiffness is sometimes relieved by rubbing the joints night and morning with Capsicum Vaseline.

Aconite.—Required in the first forty-eight hours of the disease. Febrile state. Large joints involved; hot and swollen, with shooting, cutting pains. Anguish. Thirst.

Restlessness. Painful sensitiveness, does not want to be touched.

Apis Mellifica.—Mono-articular form. Joints distended with fluid; pale; often some fluctuation and a stretched, tight feeling; burning, stinging, sticking pains; worse on motion. Parts very stiff; exceedingly sore to any pressure, with sensation of numbness.

Arnica.—Useful in the mono- and poly-articular inflammations. General bruised feeling; aggravation from motion or touch, in the evening and at night. Stiffness in the large joints. Hygroma patellæ. White swelling of the knee. Sensation of soreness in the leg.

Bryonia.—Indicated in the poly-articular variety. Sharp pain with a feeling of tension, aggravated by motion and touch; relieved by moderate pressure, rest and warmth. Acts especially on the knee and ankle joints, which are hot, swollen, with a bruised feeling. Inflammation of joints more marked than the fever would indicate. Joints very stiff with pain, as if sprained. Pale swelling of the joints, with inability to move them. Streaks of redness extend up and down the limbs from the joints. Thirst for large quantities of water.

Causticum.—Later stages. Contraction and stiffness of the tendons, especially marked in the heel and tendo-Achilles. Stitching and tearing pains. Weakness, trembling, heaviness and prostration.

Cimicifuga.—Pain in joints without appreciable lesion. Wandering pains. Hysterical hyperæsthesia of a rheumatic character.

Clematis.—Earlier stage. Pains aggravated by motion. General weakness. Rheumatic pains, with thickening of joints in the hands and fingers.

Copaiva.—Has frequently cured when the knees alone were involved.

Guaiacum.—Poly-articular form; declining stage. Contraction and stiffness of the muscles and tendons, frequently with swelling of the joints. Tearing pains. Rigidity of the joints, which are hot and swollen; they dread to move the limbs, which become thin and emaciated.

Kali Hyd.—Tearing and sticking pains in the joints, especially at night. Stiffness of the joints.

Kalmia.—Sticking, shooting, darting, tearing pains, aggravated by motion and in the evening. Bruised feeling. No swelling, no fever, but great weakness.

Mercurius.—Tearing pains, worse at night, with or without swelling. Joints puffy, of a pinkish-red color. Pains increased by warmth.

Natrum Sulph.—According to Grauvogl is a remedy which will very often be called for by the totality of the symptoms.

Phytolacca.—Feels sore and stiff from head to foot. Chronic stiffness and swelling, with loss of motion. Useful when the fibrous coverings of the joints and tendons of the muscles are involved.

Pulsatilla.—Mono and poly-articular rheumatism. Fugitive pains in various parts of the body. Lymphatic temperament. Drawing, tensive pains, with swelling and heat in the ankle and knee joints. Soft, white swelling of the knee.

Rhus Tox.—Declining stage. Acts especially on the sheaths of muscles and tendons. Bruised and sprained feeling in the large joints, relieved by continued motion and followed by weakness and stiffness of the joints. Lameness, stiffness and great weakness. Pains worse at night.

Sulphur.—A general alterative. The parts are stiff and lame. Tearing and drawing pains in the joints, etc.

Antikamnia in one-grain doses every three hours frequently gives marked relief from the unbearable pain.

CHAPTER VIII.

GONORRHŒAL AFFECTIONS OF THE EYE—GONORRHŒAL CONJUNCTIVITIS.

This most serious disease is, fortunately, quite rare, constituting only one-eighth of one per cent. of all ocular affections. Its destructive nature, however, and the imperative necessity for prompt and skillful treatment, renders it absolutely essential that the general practitioner should be sufficiently well acquainted with its symptoms and characteristics to make an early diagnosis and to institute with the smallest loss of time proper remedial measures.

Etiology.—The inflammation to which the term gonorrhœal conjunctivitis may be properly applied is always due to contagion from some source, the former theory of metastasis having no support among competent authorities.

The inoculation of the conjunctival membrane with the virus from the urethral disease may be brought about by contact with soiled handkerchiefs, towels or cloths used for bandages, from the fingers of the patient or from communication with an eye similarly affected. This may occur at any stage of gonorrhœa, but the third week is the most dangerous period, as the discharge is then most virulent.

The smallest quantity of the virus frequently suffices to set up most destructive processes, and this from either the acute or chronic form without regard to sex. Even the discharge of an old gleet may be sufficient to produce the effects. The fact remains, however, that the more noxious the virus and the larger the quantity instilled, the more serious the resulting inflammation, as a rule.

The disease occurs more frequently in men, and only one eye, usually the right, is commonly affected, by reason of the general use of the right hand. If the second eye be attacked the disease is apt to take a milder form, as the virus is less active in the later stages. The time of incubation varies from a few hours to three days, depending upon the amount and virulence of the inoculating discharge, the latter in a moist condition retaining its poisonous quality for a considerable period, but losing its activity in from thirty-six to sixty hours when dried.

Clinical History.—The first symptom usually noticed is a smarting or gritty sensation as of sand beneath the lid. The conjunctiva becomes reddened, irritable and suffused. The lids may be somewhat agglutinated in the morning with a whitish discharge. Hyperæmia of the ocular conjunctiva increases rapidly. The membrane becomes infiltrated with exudation and granular in appearance. Swelling of the lids now ensues to such a degree that they are soon closed. They are somewhat tender to touch, and there is burning in and around the eye, with neuralgic pain, photophobia and lachrymation. During the early stages the discharge is thin and acrid, and may be blood-stained. As the disease progresses the symptoms are more violent; the lids, infiltrated with exudation, become tense and shiny from the increased swelling and a livid red; the upper lid overhangs the lower; the conjunctiva is intensely red, and small hemorrhages may be noticed here and there; great chemosis is present and may overhang the cornea like a wall, constituting crater cornea; the lymphatic gland in front of the ear is swollen, and in some cases has been known to suppurate; there may be considerable fever and other constitutional disturbances.

The disease is most painful during the stage of infiltration. The great swelling of the lids makes it difficult to open them, the attempt causing much suffering. This stage attains its height in three days, when the discharge becomes purulent, creamy in color and consistency, and so profuse as to flow over the cheek in streams when the lids are opened. The discharge contains gonococci, pus cells and epithelial cells. In severe cases the pressure exerted upon the conjunctival vessels by the exudation present deprives the membrane of its blood supply, and the intense redness of excessive hyperæmia gives place to the grayish hue of anæmia. Especially is this the case when, as sometimes happens, the exudation is diphtheritic in character. Here the conjunctiva is pale, smooth and infiltrated throughout with a fibrinous exudation. The discharge is thin, gray and exceedingly acrid. This is the most dangerous form of the disease and is, fortunately, very rare. In other cases a croupous membrane may form, covering the mucous surfaces of the lids and extending upon the ocular conjunctiva. This complication is also a serious one, but in a lesser degree than the diphtheritic variety, for which it may be mistaken, although careful examination will easily differentiate between the two conditions, as the croupous membrane can be readily stripped off, leaving a reddened conjunctival surface behind, while the diphtheritic infiltration is deposited in the substance of the conjunctiva and not upon its surface.

The condition most to be dreaded in gonorrhœal conjunctivitis is ulceration of the cornea, which is of very frequent occurrence, and is due to the fact that this membrane, while largely deprived of its nutrition by the choking of the surrounding vascular supply, as a consequence of the dense conjunctival infiltration, is constantly soaked with, and its epithelial layer macerated by, an infectious discharge. As an indication of impending ulceration, opacity occurs. It may be a small speck at the centre or periphery of the cornea, or may be uniform throughout, and is immediately followed by the disintegration of the epithelium covering the affected portion, producing a destructive form of ulceration, the whole process being so rapid that a cornea may be clear one day and perforated the next.

The ulceration usually appears first at either the centre

or the margin of the cornea. If the latter, it ordinarily takes the form of a groove or furrow, which may extend peripherally in both directions, or may at once go on to perforation, which often occurs nearest the lower edge, a situation favorable to the preservation of the membrane, as here the wound may be immediately closed by the iris if the precaution has been taken to contract the pupil by the use of a solution of Eserine, preferably 1 to 200.

In all cases the cornea should be carefully examined as frequently as possible, particularly when chemosis overlaps the corneal margin, as an ulcer situated peripherally may be concealed for a time by the swollen conjunctiva. The ulceration may begin at the centre and penetrate rapidly until perforation is imminent, which will be recognized by the bulging of the membrane of Descemet, presenting a convex surface in the bottom of the ulcer. Under these conditions Atropine should be used to dilate the pupil and prevent possible entanglement of the iris in the wound, and paracentesis should at once be made to relieve pressure and in the hope that the purulent infiltration may be stayed. If spontaneous perforation supervene, it is very apt to happen at midnight, unless expedited by coughing or straining at stool. Spontaneous perforation is to be deprecated, as, aside from the fact that the lens and a portion of the vitreous may be evacuated, with the probable result of atrophy of the ball, there is great danger of extensive prolapse of the iris into the wound, a condition which invites future staphyloma. In case of such incarceration of the iris, however, it is hazardous to excise the prolapsed portion, and thus open a path for infection to the deeper structures.

In certain cases, when once purulent infiltration of the cornea has been established, no treatment seems to avail for the preservation of the membrane, and it undergoes rapid disintegration throughout its whole extent, breaking down into a yellow slough, and the eyeball may be destroyed by a consecutive panophthalmitis. Occasionally the process may be varied by the deposition of pus between the layers of the cornea, as in abscess.

The tendency to ulceration of the cornea is in proportion to the intensity of the conjunctival disease. In severe cases it may ensue by the second or third day, but it is sometimes postponed until late in the disease and then may appear without previous opacity. When it is delayed until after the tenth day the danger is lessened, as its activity is diminished, and such ulcers may heal with possible transparency. The cornea is liable to infection so long as discharge continues, though the susceptibility decreases daily.

Where pannus already exists the disease is rather beneficial than otherwise to the cornea, as it may result in the disappearance of the pannus by interference with its vascular supply.

The inflammation culminates in from five to ten days, but from four to twelve weeks may elapse before its termination.

In some cases gonorrhœal conjunctivitis is mild and may be confined to the lids and cul de sac, resembling severe catarrhal inflammation, the true condition being only revealed by microscopic examination of the discharge.

As a third stage we often have a chronic conjunctivitis with redness and thickening of the palpebral lining and elevation of its papillæ, the so-called papillary trachoma, the ocular conjunctiva being normal or somewhat hyperæmic.

The prognosis is grave. The eye may be destroyed within forty-eight hours. Eminent authorities claim that corneal trouble occurs in seventy-five per cent. of the cases, and in forty per cent. blindness ensues. Intemperate habits, bad general conditions and unfortunate surroundings diminish chances of recovery. Resultant effects vary from slight opacity to extensive staphyloma of the cornea or atrophy of the ball.

Great care must be observed by all attendants to avoid personal inoculation from squirting pus or contact with soiled linen, the discharge being still contagious when diluted up to 1–1000. In case of such inoculation the affected eye should be at once throughly cleansed with water, and Chlorine water full strength, or a two per cent. solution of Nitrate of Silver, be instilled. Either is an excellent antidote, the latter acting by its power of coagulating albumen.

Treatment.—The patient must be confined to bed and absolute cleanliness be observed. During the stage of pyorrhœa it is generally necessary to remove the discharge as often as every fifteen minutes day and night. Disinfecting solutions must be used with great frequency, the best being Merc. bichloride 1–2000, Boric Acid four per cent., and Aqua Chlorinæ ¼. Refrigeration must be employed by means of pledgets of linen fresh from the ice, and these must be constantly changed as they become warm. The use of cold applications is, however, contra-indicated when ulceration of the cornea supervenes. The pupil should be kept dilated with Atropine to prevent iritic complication, unless Eserine be indicated in threatening corneal perforation. In cases where the swelling and chemosis are extreme, scarification of the conjunctiva, canthotomy and splitting of the upper lid are advocated by many authorities. Solutions of Nitrate of Silver applied to the palpebral conjunctiva exert a great influence over the disease. Such solutions have been recommended in all strengths, from one to forty grains to the ounce, but in the writer's experience the best results have been obtained from a thirty grain solution applied once daily and immediately neutralized by a solution of Sodium Chloride. The unaffected eye must be at once isolated by strapping over it a watch crystal, great care being taken that no discharge be allowed to penetrate beneath the plaster. For this purpose it is well for the patient to lie as much as possible upon the affected side. The diet should be generous.

Acid Acetic.—Croupous form of conjunctivitis. Membrane tough and removed with difficulty.

Apis.—Great œdema, stinging pain, great photophobia and hot lachrymation, aggravated toward evening.

Argentum Nit.—This is the most useful of all remedies in this disease. The profuse purulent discharge, swelling of the lids and conjunctiva and the absence of other symptoms being its best indications.

Calcis Hypophos.—The best remedy after opacity appears, to prevent ulceration of cornea.

Hepar. Sul. C.—With ulceration of cornea and hypopyon. Great sensitiveness of lids. Intense photophobia and lachrymation. Throbbing pain. Relieved by warmth.

Kali Bich.—Croupous or diphtheritic form. Stringy discharge.

Mercurius.—More useful in decline of disease, especially for late ulceration of cornea. Discharge thin and acrid, excoriating the lids and cheek. Severe pain, worse at night. General symptoms of the remedy.

Pulsatilla.—Mild form. Profuse, bland discharge. General symptoms. Aggravation in evening. Better from fresh air.

Rhus Tox.—Thick, purulent discharge. Great swelling of cul de sac. Profuse, hot lachrymation. Restlessness. Worse about midnight.

Certain authorities have described a mild form of conjunctivitis which appears after gonorrhœal attacks, usually associated or alternating with gonorrhœal rheumatism. This form is frequently bi-lateral, resembles conjunctival catarrh and is not due to infection. Iritis may appear as a complication. Lawson describes a case of this form affecting both eyes within a week or so of gonorrhœal disease. The condition occurred with each of three gonorrhœal attacks. This case suffered severely from gonorrhœal rheumatism, each time the urethral disease appeared. The affection is exceedingly rare and should be covered by such remedies as Arg. nit., Euphrasia, Merc. and Puls.

GONORRHŒAL IRITIS.—Iritis occurring as a result of gonorrhœa is usually delayed until general infection is established, as it is commonly accompanied or preceded by rheumatism. It may be confined to one eye, but often affects both, and is believed to be due to the effects of gonococci upon the iris. It most frequently appears in the plastic form, but may be serous. A mild form, involving both plastic and serous changes has been described as peculiar to gonorrhœal infection, but this claim lacks confirmation. Rheumatic iritis may occur in the course of a gonorrhœa without articular rheumatism, but there is no evidence to prove its origin. According to Fürster, iritis may supervene whenever a gleety discharge reappears.

Clinical History.—Plastic Form.—There is hyperæmia of the conjunctiva as shown by its large, irregularly placed vessels and its brick red color; also the so-called rose pink zone about the cornea due to the injection of the deeper vessels. A little later chemosis is present. The pupil is contracted and fails to respond to the light stimulus, and the surface of the iris loses its normal appearance, becoming discolored, velvety and hazy as the result of swelling and obliteration of the normal folds. A plastic lymph is effused at the pupillary margin, and the instillation of Atropine will reveal adhesions to the lens capsule, as shown by irregular dilatation of the pupil. The aqueous humor may be hazy and there is some photophobia and lachrymation. In bad cases there may be considerable swelling and puffiness of the lids. Subjectively there is first an itching and burning followed by a more or less intense ciliary neuralgia, which may be confined to the eye or its immediate neighborhood, or may affect the entire distribution of the fifth nerve on the corresponding side of the head. The pain may be moderate during the day, but is frequently very severe at night and is usually relieved by warmth. Vision is more or less impaired, the degree depending upon the amount of lymph effused into the pupillary area and the condition of the aqueous. There may be some fever with coated tongue and other constitutional symptoms.

The tension is normal and in simple cases the eye is usually free from tenderness.

Serous Form.—In this form there is little tendency to contraction of the pupil; it may even be somewhat dilated, and the adhesions, if any, are slight and easily torn. Swelling of the iris is not present in any degree though there is some discoloration. The anterior chamber is deeper than normal, and the aqueous humor is hazy and contains floating particles of lymph, which are deposited on the posterior surface of the cornea, forming a somewhat pyramidal figure with the base downward, as the result of gravity, constituting the so-called punctate keratitis.

The deepening of the anterior chamber is due to hypersecretion of the aqueous, and the cloudiness of the latter may vary markedly, at different periods, as the result of fresh effusions. There is a tendency to increase of tension and the eye should be carefully watched, as the disease sometimes develops in the ciliary body and choroid and glaucoma may result. The symptoms are usually exceedingly mild. Vision may be considerably impaired as a result of the haziness of the aqueous and the deposits on the cornea.

The manifestations of gonorrhœal iritis are usually almost identical with those of the ordinary rheumatic form of the disease. Like the latter, it is very subject to recurrence, and there is a liability to relapse with each attack of the urethral disease.

Treatment.—Plastic Form.—The patient should be put to bed. A thick pad of cotton should be bound upon the affected side, covering not only the eye, but the whole side of the head, as warmth is usually grateful to the patient.

In some cases where severe pain is present it is necessary to replace this bandage by a bag of hot salt, which often affords relief. If, as sometimes occurs, heat should aggravate the symptoms, we have seen excellent results follow the use of the ice-bag, even in the rheumatic form of the disease. The pupil must be kept widely dilated by a mydriatic, either Atropine, four grains to the ounce, Scopolamine, Hyoscyamine or Duboisine, the latter three in a solution of $\frac{1}{200}$. Of these drugs Hyoscyamine is the most active, but must be used with caution; Atropine, the most liable to produce poisonous symptoms in young people, and Duboisine in the aged. Scopolamine should be used in all cases where glaucomatous complication is feared, as this drug, even while dilating the pupil, reduces the tension. In obstinate adhesions the chosen mydriatic may be instilled as often as every two hours if necessary, but its use must be stopped at once should toxic symptoms supervene.

The diet should be limited and selected to avoid constipation.

Bryonia.—Shooting or aching pain in and around the eye extending backward toward the occiput. Eyes feel sore on moving them in the sockets. Pains worse at night and on motion of the affected part.

Cedron.—Severe neuralgic pain in the course of the supra-orbital nerve, especially if periodic.

Cinnabar.—Particularly indicated where the pain is circum-orbital, aggravated at night.

Hepar Sul. C.—Where there is great tenderness with throbbing pain relieved by warmth. Particularly useful if hypopyon is present.

Mercurius.—Severe pains around the eye, in the forehead and temples. Throbbing and shooting, tearing or sticking in the eye. General constitutional indications for the drug—all symptoms worse at night.

Rhus Tox.—Swelling of the lids. Profuse, hot lachrymation. Chemosis. Photophobia. Restlessness. Worse about midnight. Aggravated by damp weather.

Spigelia.—Sharp, shooting pains radiating from a centre in and around the eye.

Treatment.—Serous Form.—The general care of the patient as outlined in the plastic form applies equally here. Usually the subjective symptoms are not serious. A mydriatic should be used sufficiently often to secure dilatation of the pupil, to avoid possible adhesions, and in this form Scopolamine should be the drug employed, because of the tendency to increase the ocular tension. The eye should be carefully watched for glaucomatous symptoms.

Arsenicum Alb.—Burning pain relieved by warmth. Aggravated about midnight, with restlessness and other constitutional symptoms of the drug.

Bryonia is equally useful in this form when the characteristic symptoms are present.

Gelsemium.—One of the best remedies for the serous form. Serous exudation is the best indication.

CHAPTER IX.

DISEASES OF COWPER'S AND PROSTATE GLANDS.

COWPERITIS.—Etiology.—This rarely occurs except during the course of a urethral inflammation, usually of gonorrhœal nature, appearing between the third and fourth week of the disease. It may follow instrumentation, excessive sexual indulgence, etc.

Clinical History.—Generally one gland only is involved, and by preference the left. The perinæum feels tense and painful to touch, when sitting, or even from moving the part, which may appear normal at first, but soon a small body about the size of a pea develops, somewhat movable underneath the skin, extending from the bulb backwards and terminating in front of the anus in a rounded head.

If the inflammation progresses the surrounding tissue becomes infiltrated with an inflammatory product, and the swelling will extend over the median raphé, entirely obscuring the contour of the gland; if suppuration has taken place this condition cannot be differentiated from perinæal abscess.

Treatment.—Hot fomentations, early incision, even before fluctuation appears to prevent burrowing, though this is rarely necessary, as Aconite, Cannabis sat., Sabal, Mercurius corr. will usually abort the process. Hepar sulph. and Silicea will be required later in the event of suppuration.

ACUTE PROSTATITIS.—Etiology.—It is rarely idiopathic, but usually is the result of the extension backward of a urethritis (especially of gonorrhœal nature), instrumentation, urethral injections, cauterization, or a damaged condition of the deep urethra, calculi of the prostate gland or bladder, extension of diseases of the bladder, prolonged sitting on damp, cold objects, external violence, and from the ingestion of irritating drugs, like Turpentine, Cantharides, etc.

Pathological Anatomy.—Congestion of the prostate gives rise to few symptoms, but if inflammation occurs it will become swollen, hard and œdematous, involving the surrounding tissue, often attaining from two to four times its original size.

From this condition it may return to health or a large number of minute abscesses may be developed, which are scattered rather thickly through the gland; these ultimately break down and coalesce to form one large abscess, which may burrow in many directions.

Clinical History.—When the inflammation is of slight degree there is fullness and uneasiness in the perinæum and rectum with frequent desire to urinate. These symptoms may disappear rapidly. When a urethral discharge has been the contributing cause it ceases with the advent of the disease, to be sometimes replaced by a discharge of prostatic fluid.

The pain may increase and become throbbing and lancinating in character, or a deep aching, with a sensation of fullness and soreness in the perinæum and rectum. If the finger be introduced into the rectum a hard, smooth mass, very sensitive and painful to touch, will be discovered.

There is frequent urging to stool, with pain and tenesmus, an uneasy feeling at the neck of the bladder, soreness above the symphysis pubis on deep pressure, frequent and painful desire to urinate, with straining, especially at the end of the act, sometimes accompanied by a drop ot blood, together with agonizing pains, referred to the perinæum, rectum and anus, shooting down the thighs.

These symptoms are accompanied by fever which may have been ushered in by a chill.

The prostate may yet return to its normal condition, but if suppuration takes place, chills, fever and all the symptoms of pyæmic infection will occur, and the swelling, when examined through the rectum, will feel boggy or fluctuate. As the swelling increases, diminishing still further the size of the urethra, the stream of urine becomes smaller and smaller until finally it is passed only in drops with great tenesmus, or retention follows.

The duration of the disease varies from a few days to a month.

Treatment.—Rest in bed. Hot fomentations to the perinæum. Hot rectal douches. Opium with Belladonna suppositories, though the administration of Sabal, Gelsemium, Aconite, Mercurius corr., Veratrum vir., Copaiva, Pulsatilla, Belladonna, etc., often renders their use unnecessary.

The diet must be light and consist principally of broths,

milk, matzoon, koumyss, rice, bread and milk, etc., avoiding alcohol in any form. When retention occurs withdraw the urine with a small rubber catheter as required. If an abscess develops and can be opened in the perinæum, the trouble and annoyance resulting from possible ischio-rectal fistula will be avoided. If the abscess point towards the rectum open with a punctured incision, afterwards keeping the rectum antiseptic by the frequent use of Carbolic douches. Do not discontinue treatment until the prostate is perfectly well, as there is always a marked tendency for the condition to become chronic.

**CHRONIC OR FOLLICULAR PROSTATITIS.—
Etiology.**—It is frequently the sequel of an acute gonorrhœal prostatitis, stricture of the urethra, or arises from the extension of vesical inflammation. It may commence as a sub-acute or chronic prostatitis from sexual excesses, and especially from masturbation or imperfect coitus, and undoubtedly it is also produced by dampness and cold.

This is a disease of early manhood and of middle life.

Pathological Anatomy.—The prostate may be normal in size, atrophied or swollen. Enlargement is caused by the infiltration of lymph or pus. On section the cut surface will be found spotted, red, somewhat boggy, with here and there small collections of pus, the whole organ being less firm than normal. The mucous surfaces, the sinuses of the prostate, the mucous follicles and their ducts show the most marked pathological change.

The mucous lining of the prostatic urethra is vascular and the epithelium eroded in spots. When the disease has resulted from stricture the coats are thinned, though they may be thickened, and the mouths of the prostatic gland open and pouchy.

Clinical History.—Micturition increases in frequency. It may not be perceptible or the calls may come every half hour. Often there is a slight twinge at the end of the act, and possibly a drop of blood or a little burning or tingling as the urine passes over the prostatic portion of the urethra. Micturition will be a little slow or the urine may simply drop from the penis. The pain and frequency of micturition are somewhat increased by crossing the legs, and especially on standing.

The urine is cloudy, holding in suspension small masses of muco-pus, particularly noticeable in the first ounce of urine passed, therefore have the patient void the urine in two portions for examination. The first will contain mucus in abundance, while the second may be clear. This does not always follow as the compressor urethræ muscle may be tightly or spasmodically contracted, causing the discharge to back up and empty into the bladder, mixing with the urine.

The microscope will distinguish these masses from the shreds found in gleet, revealing pus, blood corpuscles, epithelium, amyloid bodies, fatty debris and small prostatic concretions. When the prostatic fluid has been forced out by a hard stool, by a finger in the rectum or discharged as a very slight flow or moisture noticed at the meatus the addition of a one per cent. solution of Phosphate of Ammonia to the discharge will give the characteristic phosphatic crystals known as Böttcher's Crystals; but, as urethral and prostatic discharges are usually mixed, appearing as a muco-purulent discharge, we cannot always get the reaction, yet if the prostate is sensitive to pressure through the perinæum or rectum we may assume that the gland is involved. Pain may be referred to the sacrum, anus, perinæum or the inguinal region, sometimes to the neck of the bladder and end of the glans penis. This last symptom has also been caused during micturition in Prostatic Stenosis.

Chronic prostatitis causes many of the symptoms of stone in the bladder, sexual debility, premature ejaculations and physical and mental exhaustion after coitus.

They become nervous and hysterical, weak, feverish and

anæmic, and it is with the utmost difficulty that many of them can be convinced that they are not suffering from spermatorrhœa when they see the discharge from the urethra or notice a suspicious moisture at the meatus after a hard stool, even when the microscope demonstrates the absence of spermatozoa.

This condition might sometimes be confounded with Tubercular Prostatitis, but it is more chronic than the latter; it has about the same history; the absence of tuberculosis elsewhere and the microscopic examination of the secretion will clear the diagnosis.

Hypertrophy of the prostate can be diagnosed from the age of the patient, as it never occurs before the 55th to the 58th year.

Treatment.—Diet must be plain, substantial and nourishing without being too stimulating. Alcohol in all forms must be prohibited and moderation in all things advised with out-door exercise, removal to seaside or mountains, cold sponge baths in the morning, and rest in the recumbent position when possible. Sexual intercourse must be prohibited and carnal thoughts avoided. Evacuate the bowels daily by enemas.

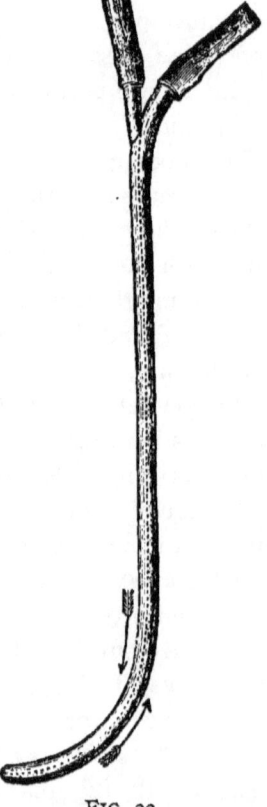

FIG. 22.

The passage of steel sounds and direct local treatment are very efficacious. The sound must be passed with the utmost gentleness and care or it will be arrested by the compressor urethræ, which is usually in a state of spasmodic contraction and is one of the many causes of the unpleasant symptoms which often arise in the disease. The passage of a full-sized sound gives great relief. Some attribute the good results derived to the *cold* sound and go further and apply cold for five minutes to the parts by means of a hollow sound, the psychrophore (Fig. 22). Others claim that the relief is due to the pressure of the sound which forces the blood out of the organ. The sound should be passed every five or eight days.

When the mucous membrane of the prostate is seriously affected, which is shown by the presence of the discharge of round masses from the lacunæ or crypts of the glands, irrigation has been used and also applications by means of the Keyes-Ultzman capillary syringe, of two or three drops of a solution of Nitrate of Silver (one to ten grains to the ounce of distilled water). These applications must not be repeated oftener than once in five days. Some authorities advise mild repeated applications of cantharidal collodion to the perinæum, painting one side up to the median raphé and keeping the patient in bed for twenty-four hours; when this has healed the opposite side is painted in like manner, the scrotum and anus being protected by absorbent cotton.

Rectal suppositories containing one and a half or two grains of Iodoform have been beneficial. One is introduced on retiring, after first cleansing the rectum with a douche.

Mercurius sol., Mercurius corr., Nitric acid, Pulsatilla, Thuja etc., will be required according to their special indications.

HYPERTROPHY OF THE PROSTATE.—Etiology.—It is a disease of advanced age never occurring before the 50th and usually not before the 60th year. Old age is its only known cause, and while strictures, cystitis, stone in the bladder, excessive venery, over-indulgence in eating and drinking, chilling of the surface, etc., may aggravate the symptoms, they never produce hypertrophy.

Pathological Anatomy.—A prostate gland, weighing

over four or six drachms, may be considered abnormal. The muscular and fibrous tissues are increased often at the expense of the glandular. In well marked cases of prostatic hypertrophy, the gland consists of little more than a circular bunch of musculo-fibrous tissue. The whole gland or either of its lateral lobes may be involved and some parts are sometimes more affected than others. Glandular enlargements or fibrous outgrowths may extend in any direction.

On section the gland will tend to pop out of its capsule. It is yellow, gray or mottled, sometimes red and more dense than normal. When the lateral lobes alone are involved the prostatic urethra is pressed together from the sides and elongated antero-posteriorly and increased in length. Symptoms may be absent, in fact a good proportion of cases of hypertrophy of the prostate are never recognized, even when the gland is much enlarged. When infiltration involves the posterior median part of the gland the condition is different and the symptoms are numerous and varied.

This portion of the gland is not covered by a capsule, consequently the growth rises from the floor of the posterior prostatic urethra and its posterior part and may project upwards like an extended lip changing the normal outlet of the bladder into a crescentic opening with its convexity upwards. The growth may also extend backwards into the bladder in shape like a large pear and somewhat pedunculated. There is frequently a bar of hypertrophied mucous membrane just behind the prostate which has been drawn up by the lateral hypertrophy. These conditions cause the long train of serious and often fatal symptoms which accompany this disease.

The hypertrophy may be confined to the posterior median portion or so-called third lobe, or the entire gland may be increased sometimes to a pound in weight. As the gland enlarges, the return circulation on its surface, through which the venous circulation of the bladder is conducted, becomes interfered with, producing passive congestion of the bladder. The dam of mucous membrane behind the prostate and the hypertrophied posterior lip not only interfere with the natural discharge of urine but prevent the complete emptying of the bladder, thus producing pathological changes and symptoms of chronic cystitis, cystic calculi, dilatation of the ureters, pyelitis, nephritis, etc.

Clinical History.—Micturition becomes more frequent, especially at night, and, as hypertrophy advances, the inclination to urinate may occur as often as every half hour. They often have to wait a short time before the flow commences; the stream comes slowly and gradually increases in force or the main stream may be projected forward while some of it at the same time dribbles or drops down perpendicularly from the end of the penis. If they strain to any extent the stream grows smaller, the effort being accompanied by some uneasiness and pain in the hypogastric region, perinæum or rectum.

The urine is sometimes small in quantity, clear and acid in reaction, but more often fetid and ammoniacal in character, containing collections of mucus, pus, phosphates, etc.

If the obstruction is not removed and inflammation extends and involves the kidneys, polyuria results; the urine will be profuse with a specific gravity of 1003 to 1006, and albumen and casts will be present. In the latter case it behooves the physician to be extremely careful as to the manner in which he performs his first instrumentation.

By some these and many other symptoms are overlooked until after a hearty meal, over-stimulation or after chilling of the lower extremities, when suddenly micturition becomes impossible, this being followed by over-distention and atony of the bladder. After producing excruciating pains this condition may possibly pass away in the following manner: after the bladder has been over-distended the neck will be pulled open and there will be an overflow and apparent relief; but this attack has added to the original lesion causing increased atony of the bladder with an aggravation of the distressing symptoms. The cystitis and retention increase as the disease progresses, the ureters, pelvis of the kidney and the kidneys themselves are involved. The walls of the bladder become thickened, sacculated, large calculi form and the urging to urinate becomes more frequent and painful. Sometimes the location of the hypertrophy makes it impossible to pass a catheter, and sudden retention can only be relieved by aspiration. This class of patients finally become thin, haggard and feverish from toxæmia, etc.

Hypertrophy of the prostate in the aged may be suspected in those who have frequent urination and digestive disturbances.

The hypogastric region must always be examined in urinary disorders when the patient is over 50 years of age to ascertain whether there is any enlargement indicating an atonic or distended bladder, as it sometimes attains the size of a fœtal head without being discovered. The urine should be passed in your presence and the effect of forced expulsion noticed. If hypertrophy is present the urinary stream will be diminished and the urine will dribble after the act.

To examine the prostate properly place the patient in the dorsal position, with the thighs flexed on the abdomen; the finger is well lubricated and introduced into the rectum, and by carrying it along the anterior wall between it and the pubes the size and character of the prostate can be easily ascertained; at the same time by bi-manual examination map out the size and condition of the bladder, which in advanced cases often contains residual urine; then carefully pass a catheter, and notice how it enters the bladder.

If catheterization is not successful, owing to hypertrophy of the posterior median lobe or dam, use a Thompson stone-searcher (Fig. 23). This instrument can be utilized to

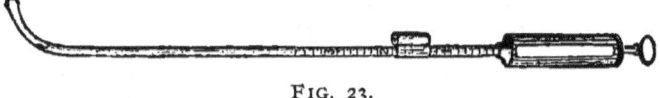

FIG. 23.

demonstrate the presence of stone often found in advanced cases, as well as to empty the bladder.

Stone can generally be detected and enlargements mapped out by turning the searcher around from side to side and drawing it backwards until the curve rests on the posterior median lip. Sometimes nothing is detected except a slight sensitiveness and enlargement of the prostate, though the most serious symptoms may be present.

Treatment.—In the milder forms of this lesion complete relief can be promised if the treatment is properly carried out, and marked amelioration in the more serious cases, which if not attended to lead to the most agonizing suffering, and ultimately to a fatal toxæmia.

Flannel must be worn at all times and the extremities guarded from exposure and sudden chilling. When arising at night to urinate, the limbs and feet must be protected by warm slippers. A warm and equable climate will be of great assistance in the treatment. Over-distention of the bladder should never be permitted; excesses in eating and drinking, over-exertion, horseback riding and sexual excesses must be prohibited. A life of moderation in all things is the only safe one.

When the urine is over-acid, causing an irritable bladder and increasing micturition, the acidity must be relieved by giving 20 grains of the Citrate of Potash in a glass of water three times daily, or by drinking plenty of Vichy. A milk diet is almost essential.

The passage every fifth day of a full-sized conical steel sound or the local application to the prostatic urethra of a solution of Nitrate of Silver (1 to 3 grains to the ounce) with the Keyes-Ultzman capillary syringe gives very good results. In the more obstinate cases, where there is atony of the bladder and retention of urine, the catheter has been relied upon to make life endurable.

Sometimes the passage of an ordinary catheter is impossible, yet a silver catheter with a long curve (Fig. 24) may

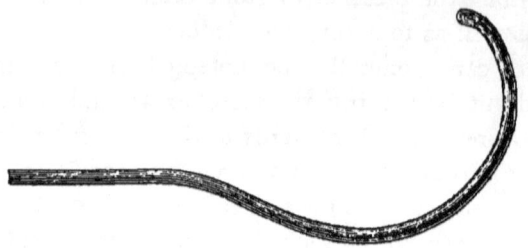

FIG. 24.

succeed; in other cases a soft, elastic catheter (Fig. 25) will

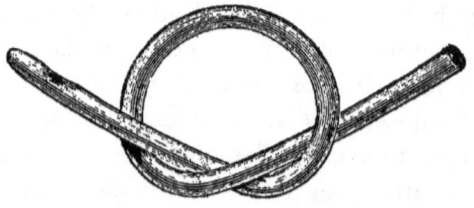

FIG. 25.

act best. It may be necessary to use Mercier's catheter, with one or two elbows (Figs. 26, 27), which compels the

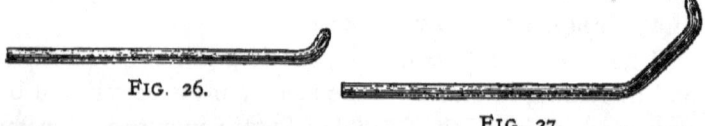

FIG. 26.   FIG. 27.

point to follow the roof of the canal and thus over-ride the dam; or an English catheter (Fig. 28) is placed for a few

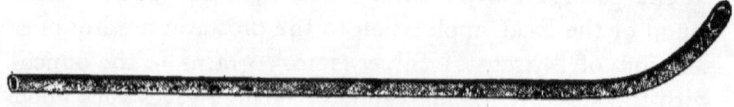

FIG. 28.

moments in hot water and moulded to an exaggerated curve, then cooled in ice water; if introduced rapidly with stylet removed, it will retain its form, and often succeeds in entering the bladder. As a last resort use the aspirator.

Always try warmth, external and internal, with the administration of Gelseminum and Aconite in alternation, and very often catheterization will not be necessary. Should the use of the catheter be decided upon, make it thoroughly aseptic, and, if the patient is to use it afterwards, instruct him as to the importance of keeping it in a solution of Boracic acid and to lubricate it before using with Carbolized Vaseline.

To insure a good night's rest when atony of the bladder exists, catheterization may be required to remove the retained urine, and may be necessary during the day.

Always place the patient in a recumbent position before introducing the catheter and always leave a little urine in the bladder, as its entire removal at the first sitting has produced shock, hæmorrhage, etc. Blood sometimes follows the withdrawal of the catheter and slight hæmorrhages may continue for some days, arising from congestion of the prostate, but this is easily checked.

Sometimes a congestion at the neck of the bladder occurs, lasting for a few days, requiring Cantharis, Aconite, or possibly the introduction into the rectum of a one or two grain Opium suppository.

Straining during micturition never facilitates the discharge and should never be encouraged, no matter how urgent the call. Dr. Hale suggests the most satisfactory method of voiding the urine for patients with hypertrophy: when ready to urinate they should grasp the penis with the hand, compress the urethra until the membranous and prostatic portions are distended with urine, thus opening the valve-like dam or bar; the grasp is then released giving full flow to the stream through the open gateway. This may have to be repeated during the act, but it lessens the irritability and insures a good stream. By following this procedure the necessity for the catheter or operation may be postponed for years. Prostatic obstructions are of such form that they can be removed by instrumentation, either through the urethra or by a supra or sub-pubic operation, or a combination of both. Within the past few years this operation has been successfully revived. Early operation is now advised, before the catheter has been used for any length of time, as it is believed that its continued and prolonged passage prevents the perfect return to usefulness of the bladder after operation.

Bottini reports 57 cases with 32 cures, 11 improvements, 12 without results and 2 deaths. He burns away the obstructing part of the gland with the thermo-galvanic cautery, introduced through the urethra. This requires a cautery plate and a cautery knife each inserted into the concavity of a short beaked catheter, with conducting wires to the plate or knife, and two water canals for cooling purposes. The plate instrument is passed as an ordinary catheter and when the point enters the bladder it is turned downward, as in sounding for stone, and gently drawn forward so as to cause the beak to press against the prostate and bring the cautery plate against the bar, when the current is turned on for a minute. This method is not free from danger and is contra-indicated when the kidneys are involved; it is best adapted to cases with persistent strangury.

Tobin has successfully removed intra-vesicular prostatic growths with an ecraseur introduced through the urethra, the loop being hooked over the projecting mass and held by the forefinger introduced through a supra-pubic opening. The advantage of this method lies in removal of only that portion of the gland which interferes with the flow of urine, leaving a smooth surface sloping into the urethra; little or no hæmorrhage occurs.

The supra-pubic perinæal operations are made according to the surgical requirements of the individual case. In 1893

Dr. J. W. White suggested castration for this class of cases, and since then many successful results have been reported, proving the operation to be as rational and justifiable as the removal of the ovaries in overgrowths of the uterus.

When dogs are castrated the prostate atrophies: autopsies have demonstrated evidence of atrophy on one side in monorchids, and complete atrophy in cryptorchids and those suffering from syphilitic sarcocele.

This operation is comparatively painless, has a low mortality and is not followed by the serious complication of supra and sub-pubic operation, yet there is sometimes a sacrifice of the sexual power, but the results of recorded cases are as satisfactory, if not more so, than those of the other and infinitely more dangerous operation, relief coming within a day or two after the operation with continued improvement.

Gelsemium, Cimicifuga, Sulphur and many other remedies may be indicated.

CHAPTER X.

DISEASES OF THE BLADDER, URETERS AND PELVIS OF THE KIDNEY.

CYSTITIS.—This is an inflammation of the walls of the bladder.

ACUTE CYSTITIS.—Attacks principally the mucous coat of the bladder in the region of the Trigon, but all the coats may be involved; it tends to pass rapidly into the chronic state.

Etiology.—Traumatism, as after child-birth, from instrumentation, etc.; introduction of an unclean catheter, over-distention of the bladder following retention, the ingestion of certain drugs as Cantharides, Turpentine, Chloride of Iron, Copaiva, etc., injections into the bladder;

extension of disease of the kidneys, ureters, prostate and urethra, especially gonorrhœa; infection in acute diseases as scarlet fever, diphtheria, etc., cold, dampness and an over-acid condition of the urine as in rheumatism, etc.

Pathological Anatomy.—The mucous membrane is red, swollen and inflamed, covered with a mucous exudate, and here and there erosions of the epithelium. The blood vessels are prominent. In severe cases the whole mucous membrane may be exfoliated as the result of over-distention or diphtheritic exudation. The muscular and serous coats also show evidence of inflammatory changes.

Clinical History.—The symptoms vary greatly in intensity. Sometimes there is only a slightly increased desire to urinate followed by an unsatisfied feeling which passes off in a few hours or days. In the graver cases there is a constant desire to urinate, inability to retain the urine, with tenesmus, burning, smarting and stinging during the act, pain in neck of bladder, at the end of the penis or in the perinæum extending down the thighs. There is soreness and uneasiness in the region of the bladder, which is quite sensitive to touch, accompanied with chill, fever and sweat.

The gonorrhœal variety, which is the most common, does not appear before the end of the second, and rarely before the end of the third week of a specified urethritis. It may vary greatly in duration and intensity. The gonorrhœal discharge lessens or ceases on the appearance of the cystitis, to return on its cure. Fever is usually absent but the tenesmus is marked, with frequent desire to urinate. The urine has a milky or bloody appearance, and contains a tenacious, stringy matter resembling thin glue. The microscope reveals pus and blood corpuscles, crystals of triple phosphates and other products of inflammation.

The other severe types of the disease arise from the introduction of bacteria by means of unclean instruments, diphtheria and traumatism.

Treatment.—Rest in bed is essential in all the severe cases. Hot fomentations and poultices to the hypogastric region and perinæum. When there is evidence of retention and percussion and palpation show an enlarged, distended bladder, the catheter should be used. When the result of cold Dulcamara will be of great benefit. If accompanied by fever and strangury Aconite, Gelsemium, Cantharis and Belladonna, the last two in alternation; Uva ursi, Terebinth, Prunus spinosa, Copaiva and Oil of Sandal-wood are frequently indicated. Triticum repens or Flaxseed tea will often be beneficial.

The strangury may require Hydrangea or Stigmata Maidis, in 20 drop doses of the θ, frequently repeated, or rectal suppositories containing one grain powdered Opium and one-fourth grain of Ext. of Belladonna.

The diet must be light, farinaceous, easy of digestion, and non-irritating; milk is the classical diet.

CHRONIC CYSTITIS rarely occurs as an idiopathic disease, but is usually secondary to some other lesion.

Etiology.—It may be the sequel of an acute cystitis, stricture of the urethra, diseases of the prostate, growths of various kinds which interfere with the normal exit of the urine, or from contiguity of tissue. It may be reflex from spinal injury or arise from sexual excesses, stone in the bladder, retention of urine, and may follow pyelitis, nephritis, pyelo-nephritis, or the introduction of bacteria into the bladder by unclean instruments. Intemperance and individual idiosyncracy often modify the disease. Acute or sub-acute attacks may be engrafted on a chronic condition at any time from cold, exposure, instrumentation, etc.

Pathological Anatomy.—The disease usually commences at the neck and fundus of the bladder involving first the mucous, but in the severe forms involving the muscular and serous coats.

In some of the old cases the membrane is pale and may present no marked pathological change to the eye when examined either at the autopsy, or during life with the Nitze electric cystoscope (Fig. 29.), which greatly facili-

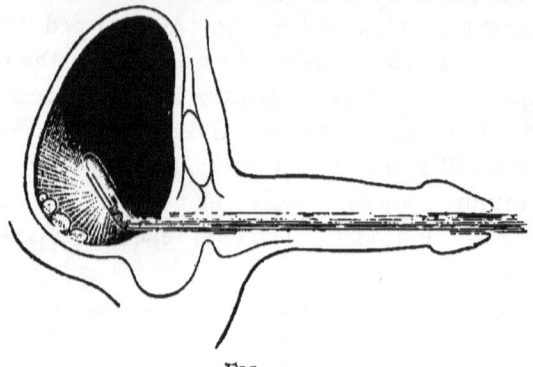

FIG. 29.

tates these examinations. This instrument is shaped like an ordinary hollow sound with a small Swan lamp fixed in the beak. It is easily passed into the bladder in the absence of stricture or other obstructions of the urethra. The special points to be observed in its use are to first wash out the bladder with a borated solution. The bladder must contain at least four ounces of clear fluid when the instrument is introduced. It requires much practice and persistence to appreciate the normal and abnormal conditions revealed by the cystoscope. It may be necessary to use anæsthesia, local or general, to facilitate its introduction, but as a rule the parts are not over-sensitive and anæsthesia is seldom required.

The membrane, however, is generally swollen and less firm than normal, with congestion and extravasation of blood in spots. The vessels are enlarged and varicosed, filled with dark blood, with here and there erosions and ulcerations of the mucous coat, its surface being covered with glairy mucus or a chocolate-colored fluid, composed of broken-down cells, Ammoniaco-Magnesian Phosphates, etc.

The ureters may be inflamed, dilated, and contain muco-pus, which may completely occlude them. The pelvis of the kidney and even the kidney tissue may present evidence of inflammation and compression from retained urine. Such pathological changes will also account for the polyuria sometimes present in this form of the disease.

The cellular tissue of the vesical wall may be infiltrated with inflammatory products that undergo retrograde metamorphosis and finally breaks down, or the mucous membrane may be found ulcerated, exposing the muscular coat. The muscular coat may be hypertrophied, with or without dilatation; sometimes contraction of the viscus occurs, especially from the irritation of an acid urine, but usually it is dilated from an atonic condition of the bladder. The muscular coat may be atrophied here and there, allowing the development of pouches, whose walls are composed of membranous and serous coats only; the muscles may, on the other hand, stand out like large bands or cords, which are of a deep bluish-red or purple color. These muscles are sometimes eaten through and project as stumpy, ulcerated masses into the cavity of the bladder. Sometimes ulceration between the muscular bands occurs, which may perforate the peritonæum and adjacent parts.

When the disease is of long standing and the walls of the bladder have become dilated and thinned, that organ will be found sacculated, sometimes containing from 2 to 8 pints of alkaline, foetid, chocolate-colored urine.

Clinical History.—This will vary greatly with the cause and duration of the disease.

The exciting cause will govern not only the severity of the disease, but also the persistence of this or that symptom or set of symptoms, and will vary from a moderate case with slightly increased frequency of micturition, slight uneasiness and burning during the act and an uncomfortable feeling referred to the sub-pubic region, to one in which the desire to urinate is constant and attended with the most agonizing burning pains and tenesmus.

The general health is impaired by the retention in the circulation of urea, the diseased condition of the kidneys preventing its proper elimination, as well as the introduction into the system of bacteria and their ptomaines developed in the diseased bladder.

This systemic toxæmia is recognized by the following symptoms: great prostration, emaciation, weakness, thirst, hectic fever, restlessness, constipation, sometimes diarrhœa, and finally, if the case is to terminate fatally, by a low or typhoid state, with dry tongue, irritable stomach, uriniferous breath, delirium and coma rapidly closing the scene (urinary fever).

The condition of the urine varies with the duration of the disease and the pathological conditions present. It may be mildly acid, turbid or milky, containing pus, albumen and epithelium, but as retention becomes more persistent the urea gradually decomposes into Carbonate of Ammonia which attacks the mucous membrane, adding still further to the existing pathological changes. The retained urine is alkaline from the ammoniacal decomposition and neutralizes the acid urine as it flows from the ureters. The pus and mucus are converted into a yellow, stringy and tenacious mass, which may be drawn out into long strings without parting, and containing in its meshes ammoniaco-magnesian and amorphous phosphates, blood corpuscles, etc. In the advanced state of the disease the urine becomes chocolate-colored, of pungent and ammoniacal odor, micturition becomes more frequent and agonizing, especially towards the end of the act, with pain referred to the sacrum, lower part of the abdomen, penis, back and thighs. If atony and dilatation are present to any extent the tenesmus will increase in violence and dribbling of the urine from overflow occurs; the quantity passed at each urination is only the excess accumulated between the acts. The overdistended bladder may sometimes extend as high up as the umbilicus.

These cases all tend to grow worse unless placed under proper care. If the cause can be removed they may be cured; when this is not possible great relief often follows the proper treatment.

Treatment.—Fatigue and exposure of all kinds must be avoided and flannel underclothing should be worn at all times. The calls of nature must receive prompt attention to avoid overdistending the bladder. The diet must be plain and the larger the quantity of milk, skimmed milk, koumyss, matzoon or malted milk ingested and the less undigestible food eaten, the more satisfactory will be the results.

Remove the cause if possible. If the urine is over acid an alkali is indicated. Where there is evidence of bacteriological growth Salol should be administered. This drug is decomposed in the system into Carbolic and Salicylic acids, and is secreted by the kidneys, acting as a direct local application to the diseased parts. If diseases of the kidneys exist it must not be administered in large doses, as toxic symptoms sometimes follow its use. Sodium salicylate and Boracic acid act in the same manner as local disinfectants.

The best and most satisfactory results are obtained by washing out the bladder with a Marcy double current catheter (Fig. 30) with fountain syringe, or, better yet, by

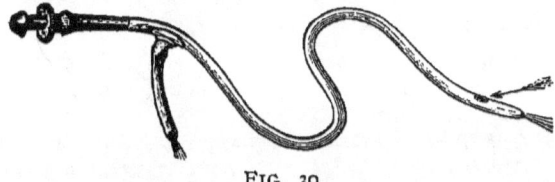

FIG. 30.

Skene's apparatus, which consists of a soft rubber catheter joined to a piece of soft rubber tubing by means of a small glass tube, the whole being about two feet long; a small glass funnel is inserted into the end of the tubing, completing the apparatus. It is used as a catheter to empty the bladder of the urine; after this is done the washing out is accomplished by pouring the solution to be used into the funnel, which is raised high enough to allow it to flow by gravity into the bladder; the funnel is then lowered to permit the fluid to escape. This process is repeated as often as necessary, using any desired quantity and pressure.

It is of the greatest importance to exclude air from the bladder; this can be accomplished by the patient retaining a small quantity of urine in the bladder; when ready for the operation introduce the catheter and remove the urine or allow the patient to urinate through it, and the catheter and tube will remain filled. If the bladder is empty the catheter should be filled before introducing it. Continue the washing until the fluid comes away clear. Great care should always be taken to wash the catheter in hot water, keeping it, when not in use, in a saturated solution of Boracic acid, and lubricate it before introduction with Carbolized Vaseline or soap and water. Always leave some of the fluid in the bladder after the first few washings, gradually reducing the quantity each time. In many cases it is unwise to commence irrigations at once or to repeat them too frequently. It must be remembered that in chronic cases of vesical disorders the bladder does not at first tolerate liquids of low specific gravity, hence the necessity of increasing their density. Dr. Gouley recommends the following:

℞ Hydrarg. Chlor. Corr., ... gr. v.
Ammonii Chlor., ... gr. xx.
Spts. Gaultheriæ, ... fl. ʒss.
Acid. Boracic., ... ʒi.
Glycerinum, ... fl. ʒviii.
M.

Sig. To ½ fluid ounce of this solution add seven fluid ounces of warm water (110° F.) and two and a half fluid ounces of Hydrogen peroxide. This ten-ounce solution is sufficient for four washings.

The following solutions give good results: Bichloride of Mercury 1 to 5000, to 20,000, Nitrate of Silver 1 to

500, to 2000, Permanganate of Potash 1 to 250, Carbolic Acid 1 to 500, Hydrogen peroxide 15 vol. ¼ to full strength, Pyrozone 3 %, ¼ to full strength, Borolyptol ¼ to full strength, or solutions of Borax, Sodium chloride, Boracic acid, Ernesty's Aqueous, Hydrastis, a teaspoonful to the quart of warm water. The Borax solution is believed to be the best. The above solutions should be used at a temperature of 90 to 100° F. Irritation of the bladder and the frequent calls to urinate may be palliated by the instillation into the deep urethra of a few drops of a 4 per cent. solution of Cocaine.

In this disease we obtain the most gratifying results from remedies even without local treatment. The most important of these are Chimaphila, Eucalyptus, Copaiva, Berberis, Prunus spinosa, Kava, Thuja, Uva ursi, Terebinth, Pichi, Populus, Pulsatilla, and Grindelia.

NEURALGIA OR IRRITABILITY OF THE BLADDER.—This is due to abnormal conditions at the neck of the bladder in both the male and female; in the male the prostatic sinus around the seminal ducts is congested and irritated.

Etiology.—It is frequently observed to be associated with or caused by some perverted sexual habit or fancies, a concentrated condition of the urine, a gouty or strumous diathesis, or by reflex conditions, as stone in the bladder, prostatic disease, rectal, uterine or ovarian lesions and tænia, vegetations, growths or congenital or acquired contractions at the meatus urinarius. In the female these growths can be removed by the button-hole operation, or more easily by snipping them off, at the same time taking a portion of the membrane and cauterizing with Nitric acid or Pyrozone 25 per cent.

Clinical History.—Its development is slow, but it may commence with an inflammatory condition and disappear with it. There is a frequent desire to urinate, usually without burning, smarting or tenesmus, but these may be present. The micturition is not at all times satisfactory, and the desire may return in a few minutes, especially if the patient is worried, mentally depressed, or exposed to a damp, cold atmosphere. On the other hand, if pleasantly engaged or somewhat exhilarated by drink, hours may pass before the least inconvenience or desire is experienced; sleep is not disturbed.

The urine may be passed slowly; sometimes there is a short wait before the act, caused by spasm of the muscles of the membranous urethra, at other times it will start with a spurt. The urine is clear and free from pus, epithelium or mucus, acid in reaction and contains crystals of amorphous phosphates, urates and oxalates.

Erections may be frequent or absent with some uneasiness around the scrotum, and especially the rectum; possibly a little irritation is experienced at night and sometimes dull, dragging pains with disturbance of the bowels.

The passage of a full-sized sound will give evidence of spasmodic constriction in both the membranous and prostatic portions of the urethra; it may cause faintness, desire to urinate or seminal emissions. On its removal a trace of blood may sometimes be noticed on the instrument, but the passage of the sound usually gives marked relief for a few days although a slight burning may accompany the next act of micturition.

Treatment.—Remove the cause. Improve the general health and morale of the patient. Recommend outdoor employment. The passage of a full-sized steel sound every fourth day has cured many cases. Applications to the prostatic urethra, by means of Taylor's syringe, of two or three drops of a solution of Nitrate of Silver, one to two grains to the ounce of water, are sometimes required. The condition, however, may be relieved by the following remedies: Nux vomica in the gouty and strumous; Belladonna, Ferrum acet. or Ferrum phos. if there is congestion; Rhus aromatica, Hyoscyamus, Buchu, Equisetum, etc.

INCONTINENCE OF URINE.—This is of frequent occurrence and may be the result of many diseased conditions; it is a symptom and not a disease. It is frequently met with in young children and women and may be caused by a hearty meal late at night, the drinking of much water before retiring, neglect on the part of the parent to see that the child urinated before going to bed. It may be reflex from a narrowed prepuce, the accumulation of smegma behind the glans penis, or adhesion of the hood of the clitoris.

It is often the first symptom of Bright's disease, it may indicate stone in the bladder, and worms either in the rectum or vagina, or arise from spinal irritation, diminished activity in the vesico-spinal centre in the lumbar part of the cord, epileptic conditions, chorea of the bladder which may be accompanied by other choreiform movements.

Clinical History.—This condition occurs at night and is usually due to an exaggerated action of the muscular coat of the bladder. The compressor urethræ is off guard and the contents of the bladder are discharged when this muscle is affected by loss of power.

Enuresis is not necessarily continuous, it may be intermittent or occur only from exposure to cold or fright.

In the adult it is usually the result of retention of urine and an overflow from the bladder, but it may be due to a want of power in the muscular coat of the membranous urethra, hypertrophy of the bladder or irregular development of the prostate gland so that the bladder overflows when filled beyond a certain point.

Treatment.—Remove the cause if possible. Avoid eating hearty meals and drinking late in the evening. Children afflicted with enuresis should be awakened and taken up during the night to urinate, and above all don't scold or whip them. Keep a light burning in the room to lessen the depth of sleep. When the urine is over-acid give an alkali, and if ammoniacal Benzoic acid will be indicated.

Remedies: Causticum, Pulsatilla, Gelsemium, Hyoscyamus, Rhus aromatica, Nux vomica, Stramonium, Equisetum, Triticum repens, Terebinth, Cina, Santonin, Agaricus, Cimicifuga, etc. Phenacetin and Antipyrine, may be administered in doses of 1 to 5 grs. at bed-time to relieve vesical irritability either in hypertrophy of the muscular walls or atony of the compressor urethræ; this allows the urine to be retained for some hours.

Electricity has been recommended with varying results. With the galvanic current a broad, flat pad attached to the negative pole is placed over the lower dorsal or lumbar region, and a button electrode connected with the positive pole is applied at the perinæum, and a mild current given daily or every second day. Others apply the positive pole to the lumbar region and the negative over the bladder or in the urethra by means of a small urethral electrode. The Faradic current has also been used to advantage. Brandt reports a number of cases in females cured by massage of the bladder, administered as follows: the patient stands leaning slightly forward with the hands against the wall, a rapid springy percussion is made down both sides of the spine with the closed fists. Then beginning at the lumbar region down over the buttocks with the open hands, stroke the parts downwards three or four times. The patient then assumes the dorsal position, the hands of the operator with the ulnar surfaces approximated and the finger tips directed towards the pubes; the fingers are pushed deep into that region by the side of the bladder as if to grasp it, and a vibratory movement is made with each hand as if the operator was about to remove the organ. This is repeated three times. The index finger of the left hand is then introduced into the vagina and flexed obliquely so as to partly encircle the neck of the bladder. The right hand grasps the wrist to make it firm, the index finger is now made to vibrate against the neck, pressing it firmly against the pubes. This is done three or four times and repeated with the right hand. The knees and heels are brought together and the patient raises the pelvis and supports herself on heels and shoulders; this is repeated as before. The hands of the operator are then placed on the inner side of the knees, the limbs forced apart while the patient resists the movement, then the operator tries to prevent her closing them. This is repeated four or five times, and finally the tapotement of the lumbar region is again performed. In children and males the finger is introduced into the rectum.

When due to overflow from retention the treatment is the same as advised for that condition.

RETENTION OF URINE.—This is a symptom which is classed as a disease, but is simply an indication of voluntary or involuntary retention of the urine. Voluntary retention is practiced by children at play, young girls and women from inconvenience or procrastination. In time it may lead to atony of the muscular coat of the bladder and true retention.

True retention may be due to overdistention of the bladder from paralysis of its muscular coat, inflammation and strictured condition in any part of the urethra, spasm of the compressor urethræ, congestion, inflammation and growths of the prostate, or from a general blunted sensibility, as in delirium, coma, etc.

Clinical History.—This condition sometimes appears suddenly after excesses or exposure, or insidiously from growths of the prostrate gland, etc. When long continued there will be dribbling of urine, from overflow, with straining and inability to urinate, accompanied by much pain in the bladder and neighboring parts, great anxiety and general distress. Palpation will reveal a distended bladder filling up the hypogastric region, extending sometimes to the umbilicus, with flatness on percussion. If a finger of the disengaged hand is placed in the rectum fluctuation can easily be obtained. If not relieved the ureters and kidneys are soon involved, resulting finally in coma and death.

Differentiation of this condition from suppression of the urine is easy. In suppression there is no enlargement of the bladder, as shown by the negative physical signs: no tumor, no fluctuation and no desire to urinate on pressing over the region of the bladder.

Treatment.—Remove a portion of the urine at once, if possible, with a perfectly aseptic soft rubber catheter; if unsuccessful try hot fomentations to the hypogastrium, perinæum and genitals, with rectal enemas of warm water; also allow water to flow from a faucet in their hearing. If the retention is the result of spinal disease and there is loss of the knee-jerk, as in tabes dorsalis, general paralysis, polyneuritis or injuries of the spinal cord, the urine may be expelled by pressure over the supra-pubic region without the use of the catheter.

Remedies—Nux vomica, Gelsemium, Belladonna, Secale, Opium, Hyoscyamus, Cantharis, Aconite, Cubeba, Copaiva, Terebinth, Apis, Pichi, Cannabis sativa, etc., as indicated. If these means fail use the aspirator or trocar, then seek and treat the cause of the retention.

STRANGURY OR VESICAL TENESMUS.—This consists of an uncontrollable, agonizing straining and contraction of the neck of the bladder. It occurs as a symptom of many acute diseases and may be of neuralgic or inflammatory origin.

Treatment.—The electro-static current applied to the spine and hypogastrium has given immediate relief. Camphor, in repeated doses, usually acts satisfactorily; Cantharis, Belladonna or Hydrangea; and in the *female* Copaiva, Eupatorium perfoliatum, and possibly Apis or Capsicum may be required.

CHAPTER XI.

STONE IN THE BLADDER.

VESICAL CALCULUS.—A vesical calculus is a concretion of variable size formed by an aggregation of some of the solid constituents of the urine which have been precipitated in more or less crystalline form. The crystalline substances are arranged with some degree of regularity, and are held together by a albuminoid frame-work derived from the mucus secreted by the urinary tract. The stone usually has its origin in a nucleus which may be a large crystal, bit of tenacious mucus, blood clot, or some foreign body accidentally or intentionally introduced into the bladder. Upon this nucleus urinary solids are deposited, the diathesis of the patient and local conditions within the bladder determining their character and quantity. A calculus is classified according to its composition, if compound taking the name of the ingredient forming its bulk. Uric acid, Oxalate of Lime, and Phosphates, in the order named, are the most frequent constituents of stone, but concretions of Xanthin, Cystin and Indican, though rare, are occasionally found. It is quite usual to find a stone composed of more than one ingredient; thus a Uric acid nucleus may be surrounded by a lamina of Oxalate of Lime and the whole incrusted with a layer of Phosphates. There is great variety in size and weight, from a small gravel of a few grains to a mass weighing one or two pounds. The contour will depend largely upon the shape of the nucleus and effects of friction, for should there be more than one stone, or a single stone undergo spontaneous fracture, the multiple calculi or the fragments will show polished facets from mutual attrition. The surface of a calculus is usually rough, particularly in the Oxalate of

Lime variety, its knobbed or beaded appearance giving it the name of "mulberry calculus." The Uric acid stone is the most frequently met with, occurring, according to Roberts, in fifty per cent. of all cases. It is hard, usually brownish and reddish-brown in color, and does not attain great size, except when its bulk is increased by the deposit of phosphatic encrustations induced by the irritation which its presence causes. The Oxalate of Lime variety is small, round and very hard, and does not readily yield to crushing operations. Phosphatic stones, usually found in old men, are large, grayish-white in color, chalky in consistency, and friable.

Etiology.—Age is an important etiological factor in the production of stone, the greater number being found at the extremes of life. In childhood and old age the anatomical arrangement of the genito-urinary tract is most favorable for its development. Hereditary gout and rheumatism furnish predisposing causes for formation of calculi. Life under poor hygienic conditions, which induce mal-assimilation of food and interfere with its proper oxidation, favors the development of diatheses, which form a ground-work leading to the production of stone. There is no evidence that the continued ingestion of drinking water strongly impregnated with inorganic salts can *per se* be capable of producing a calculus. Any condition which causes retention of urine and its consequent decomposition favors the formation of concretions. Among these conditions are enlarged prostate, tight stricture, long and adherent prepuce, and tight meatus in boys.

Symptoms.—Usually the first symptoms produced by the presence of a calculus are pain and increased micturition with more or less tenesmus. Pain varies in intensity and character, sometimes being dull, aching or a heaviness in the perinæum; again sharp, lancinating or burning. It is seldom felt in the bladder, but often referred to the end of the penis or to the under surface of the urethra, a short distance posterior to the meatus. It is most marked during or at the completion of the urinary act, and is very severe in character. The constant contact of the stone with the already inflamed vesical neck produces an irritation which finally becomes a marked inflammation. Lying on the back, particularly with the hips elevated, causes the stone to roll backward, and is usually a grateful position. Micturition occurs less frequently at night, but very often during the day when the patient is subjected to the jerking occasioned by riding or walking. This state of affairs is reversed in the patient with an enlarged prostate, who is obliged to urinate often at night, but is rather free from that annoyance when his mind is busily engaged during the day. The effect of motion, if it be violent, is to cause a traumatism of the already inflamed bladder walls giving rise to hæmaturia, from the mere presence of blood in the urine to vesical hæmorrhage. Reflex pains are felt in different parts of the body; testicles, hips, thighs and soles of the feet. If the stone is small it often rolls over the internal orifice of the urethra, and with a ball-valve action stops the stream at the height of the urinary act. This stoppage causes pain and straining, but both are usually relieved when the patient changes his position, particularly when he lies down. Priapism is another symptom noticed particularly in young boys, often giving rise to masturbation.

The symptoms above described constitute strong presumptive evidence of the existence of a vesical calculus, but its presence is only positively determined when a metal sound is introduced into the moderately distended bladder and made to touch the stone, when the characteristic "click" is heard and a sensation imparted to the hand. This procedure, called "sounding," should be dignified as an operation, and the greatest care should be observed in the preparation of patient and instruments.

Should there be an acute outburst of vesical symptoms,

and it is usually at such a period that the physician sees the patient, rest in bed, diluents and remedies should be used until a quiescent state of the bladder is obtained. We have seen serious consequences follow the disregard of this very natural precaution, for the reaction following this manipulation, particularly in old men, is often very severe. Again, the errror is made often in the opposite direction and a patient treated for the indefinite condition, "catarrh of the bladder," stone never being suspected.

Before the operation the urine is carefully examined, and, according to its acidity, alkalinity or concentration, some pure water like Poland or Clysmic, or a mineral water like Lithia, should be given in sufficient quantities to change the characteristics of the urine. If it be fœtid the internal administration of Salol or Boracic acid will tend to render it antiseptic. When sounding is to be performed the patient is placed in the dorsal position, thighs and legs extended, upon a table or couch.

Anæsthesia is usually not necessary for the preliminary sounding, as the stone may be discovered with but little difficulty. But if the patient is old, and there is a probability that manipulation will not be readily borne, preparations should be made so that if stone is discovered an operation for its removal may take place immediately following the sounding.

The greatest care should be observed in the preparation of instruments which are to pass into the bladder. They should be surgically clean and all strong antiseptic solutions removed before introduction into the bladder by dipping them in sterilized water. Very annoying urethritis is often produced by the action of a strong germicide applied to the urethral mucous membrane from an instrument dipped in the same. The bladder should contain four or five ounces of fluid. A Thompson searcher is introduced and passed toward the posterior wall of the bladder to the fundus, which is the most frequent situation of stone. The instrument is now withdrawn a short distance at a time, being rotated from side to side, so that its beak describes an arc of a circle and touches the base and lateral walls of the bladder at each turn. This manœuvre, somewhat varied, is performed many times. In a patient with enlarged prostate the existence of the post-prostatic pouch is to be remembered, and during the withdrawal of the instrument, when its beak is about the centre of the bladder, it is rotated through half a circle and made to explore this cavity. If these manœuvres are followed by negative results, some water is drawn off, gentle efforts make the bladder partially collapse; the patient may also be made to stand while the water is flowing off, when the stone often falls forward against the searcher.

A stone may be present but not discovered because of its being encapsulated by the walls of the bladder, or its surface covered with blood or mucus so that it gives no sound when touched. Again mistakes may be made by mistaking tumors encrusted with phosphates for stone, or the stone itself may be of such light specific gravity as not to give sufficient striking contact to be perceived by the sound. The old rule in surgery was never to operate for stone unless its presence could be determined when the patient was placed upon the table, no matter how recently it had been demonstrated.

If the stone is found, contact of the beak of the searcher with its surface will tell whether it is rough or smooth, and the sound emitted by striking it will be sharp and clear if Uric acid or Oxalate of Lime, and dull if phosphatic. Two stones are present, if, when the patient is quiet, rotating the searcher from side to side produces a separate click on each side. The size of a stone may be often determined by passing a finger into the rectum and palpating between the searcher and finger. Again the searcher is introduced and its beak turned toward the side of the bladder where the stone was discovered and quietly rotated in that direction while being withdrawn. When the stone is struck the collar of the instrument is pushed against the meatus, the tapping is continued, and when the click is no longer heard the end of the stone is reached and the distance between the collar of the searcher and the meatus will represent one of the diameters of the stone. After completion of the search the bladder should be washed with Thiersch's solution.

Non-Operative Treatment of Stone.—The so-called "solvent treatment," the internal administration of certain drugs and the injection into the bladder of substances, all for the object of producing a chemical disintegration of the calculus, has from lack of success fallen into disuse. This method has existed from ancient times and has an interesting history, which is even now occasionally added to by the introduction of a new drug which in the laboratory seems to possess the requisite qualites, but which practically fails. Much can be done as a matter of prophylaxis. A patient having an attack of renal colic should be taken in hand at once and such methods employed to rid him of the tendencies which ultimately succeed in producing a calculus. Attention to diet is of first importance. Consideration must be given to the peculiarities of each patient. More frequently trouble arises from indulgence in the starchy, saccharine and oleaginous constituents of diet. Bread should be partaken of sparingly and lean meats, poultry, game, fresh fish, oysters and eggs should form the basis of the diet. The succulent vegetables, such as lettuce, spinach, celery and fruits, may be taken with safety. Many beneficial effects follow the use of large quantities of pure water, like Poland, Clysmic, Bedford, Bethesda, etc. Milk is an excellent article of diet for such patients and may be given plain, skimmed, with lime water, peptonized or aerated with any of the carbonated mineral waters and can be made to suit almost any phase of the patient's condition. Alcohol should, if possible, be interdicted or limited to white wine or a light claret. Exercise in the open air, not to be carried to the point of excessive fatigue or profuse sweating, should be advised. At this time remedies selected according to the diathesis possessed by the patient in conjunction with dietetic and hygienic precautions will often produce very happy results.

The Operative Treatment of Stone.—The factors influencing the choice of an operation depend upon (1) age and general condition of the patient; (2) state of the genito-urinary tract; (3) the size and composition of the stone.

The methods at our command are supra-pubic lithotomy, perinæal lithotomy, median and lateral and litholapaxy. From exhaustive statistics, considering age, Cabot has shown that in children, from infancy to fourteen years, there is little to choose between litholapaxy and lateral lithotomy, slight advantage being in favor of the former, the supra-pubic operation being more dangerous than either. In adult life the results decidedly favor litholapaxy, the danger of cutting operations increasing with age. In old age the rate of mortality is overwhelmingly in favor of litholapaxy, an operation extremely well borne at this time of life, notwithstanding the high mortality attending the performance of any variety of lithotomy. When, however, the calculus is complicated with a tumor of the bladder, when it is encysted, or too large or too hard to be crushed, lithotomy must be practiced. Litholapaxy is particularly contra-indicated when from a deep, unyielding stricture or enlarged prostate the instruments could only be passed by using a dangerous amount of force; also when there is reason to suspect that the nucleus of the stone is a foreign body not amenable to the lithotrite. The supra-pubic or high operation, a procedure of much value, had received little attention from recent surgeons, but owing to the efforts of Prof. Wm. Tod Helmuth it has been happily revived. It is best adapted to large, hard or encysted stones. It is well indicated in old men, in whom litholapaxy is impracticable. Also when it is expedient to remove a calculus and operate upon an enlarged prostate at the same time.

For a perineal lithotomy the patient is placed upon his back upon a narrow table which has been covered with a rubber cloth, so arranged that it will convey the blood and solutions to a pail placed beneath. At least three assistants are required, one to administer the anæsthetic, another to steady the knees and at the same time hold the staff the third to use the sponge. If available it is well to use one of the several varieties of retentive apparatus to secure the knees and hold them apart. The rectum having been previously emptied, the bladder washed out with a Boro-Salicylic solution (Salicylic acid 1 part, Boracic acid 6 parts and water 500 parts) the pubes and perinæum are shaved, scrubbed and douched with a sublimate solution. The legs and thighs are thoroughly cleansed and wrapped in antiseptic towels. The rule in surgery that no matter how recently the stone has been discovered its presence must be demonstrated at the time of the operation is to be remembered The fact that the staff strikes it when introduced shows the presence of the stone and also that the instrument has entered the bladder. About eight ounces of warm Boracic solution are injected into the bladder, the staff (Fig. 31) introduced and passed to an assistant, who

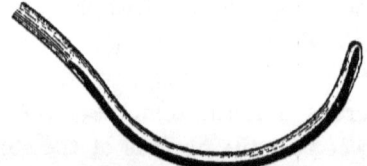

FIG. 31.

holds its handle vertically from the body and bringing its concavity firmly against the pubic arch. The operator, seated in a chair of convenient height, is now ready for the operation.

If lateral lithotomy is intended the operator steadies the integument of the perinæum with his left hand and with the lithotomy knife (Fig. 32) makes an incision from a

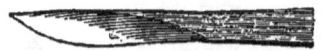

FIG. 32.

point to the left of the raphé, an inch and a quarter in front of the anus, downward and outward to a point about midway between the anus and tuberosity of the ischium, but nearer the tuberosity. Care should be taken not to make the upper portion of this incision too deep, so as to avoid wounding the bulb. The superficial structures being divided the surgeon introduces the left forefinger into the wound and feels for the staff. When found the fingernail is made to rest against the groove and the knife introduced. When certain that the point of the knife is in the bottom of the groove, it is pushed along until it enters the bladder. This fact is known by the gush of fluid which follows the opening of the viscus. The wound is enlarged by increasing the incision somewhat in a horizontal direction so as to cut through the thickest portion of the lateral lobe of the prostate. The right forefinger is now introduced into the bladder through the wound and the search made for the stone. If the incision is too small it may be further enlarged by use of the probe-pointed bistoury (Fig. 33). When the stone is located the staff is

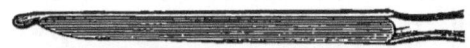

FIG. 33.

withdrawn and the lithotomy forceps (Fig. 34) introduced, using the finger as a guide. They are opened in the bladder, rotated and closed, when the stone will usually be found in their grasp. It must now slowly, and with a side to side movement, be withdrawn from the bladder in the axis of the pelvis. If possible fragmentation is to be avoided, but should it crumble in the jaws of the forceps, the several fragments must be removed by the use of a syringe and tube. There is usually some hæmorrhage. Vessels in sight can be caught and ligated with catgut, hot water will usually stop oozing; should it continue a square of antiseptic muslin is perforated in the centre, through the opening of which a stout rubber tube is passed and secured so that about three inches of it project, this makes

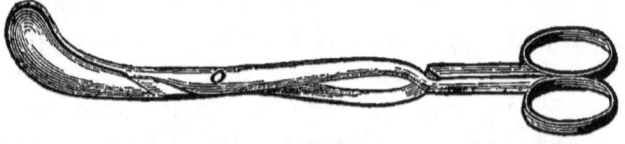

FIG. 34.

the "chemise canula." The point of the tube is passed into the bladder and the umbrella portion is tightly packed with antiseptic gauze so as to make firm, equable pressure. The wound is covered with iodoform gauze. The skin in the immediate vicinity is anointed with iodoformized vaseline to prevent irritation from urine. The patient is placed upon pads of wood wool or salicylated paper. All dressings are to be changed when soaked with urine. Drainage tube is not to be used unless the urine is very foul.

Median Lithotomy.—The patient is placed in the lithotomy position as before, and the staff introduced. The left index finger in the rectum locates the staff at the apex of the prostate. A straight bistoury with a double cutting point is made to transfix the perinæum exactly in the raphé, half an inch in front of the anus and carried directly inwards to the groove in the staff at the point where the instrument is felt in the rectum. The knife is advanced slightly so as to enter the urethra and slightly incise the apex of the prostate. The knife is now made to cut forward and divide the membranous urethra. It is withdrawn cutting its way out along the raphé, making an incision about one and a quarter inches long. A straight-grooved director is introduced and the staff withdrawn. The wound should now be dilated with the fingers and the stone extracted. Should sufficient dilatation not be obtained in this way the opening may be enlarged by making incisions downward into the prostate. This operation is only intended for small stones.

Supra-Pubic Lithotomy.—The anterior surface of the bladder is not covered by the peritoneum; the latter is reflected from the former posterior to the point of continuity of the urachus with the viscus. It is attached firmly to the summit and anterior surface of the bladder, but loosely to the abdominal wall at the point of reflection, thus enabling it to accommodate itself to the various changes in size and position of the bladder. A space exists immediately behind and above the symphysis pubis not covered by peritoneum, which, by distending the rectum and bladder, can be increased to a considerable degree. The usual preparations for lithotomy having been observed the patient is etherized and the pubic region shaved and made antiseptic. A soft rubber bag or "colpeurynter" is introduced into the rectum. The bladder having been irrigated, seven or eight ounces of the Boro-Salicylic solution are carefully injected and allowed to remain, the penis being tied with a piece of rubber drainage tube. Filling of the bladder requires some caution, as rupture of that viscus has occurred during this procedure. The rectal bag is now filled with from fifteen to eighteen ounces of water. Some operators prefer to dispense with the rectal bag, placing the patient in Trendelenberg's position, when the bladder by its own weight separates the pre-vesical fold from the pubes.

Bristowe has found from experience that the bladder is lifted up easier and more thoroughly with air. By his method air is injected with a syringe, which has between the bulb and injecting nozzle a glass tube filled with a filter of sterilized cotton. Either of the above methods having been employed an incision is made exactly in the median line, begining about three inches above and stopping at the symphysis. A layer of loose tissue containing fat will have to be separated before the bladder wall comes into view. A small transverse incision is made in this tissue at the inferior angle of the wound and the forefinger introduced and pushed upwards, carrying before it the reflection of the peritoneum. The venos plexus at the bottom of the wound should be pushed aside or divided between double ligatures, as it sometimes gives rise to troublesome hæmorrhage. The bladder may be now secured by the introduction with a curved needle of stout silk ligatures, one on either side of the proposed incision. The pre-vesical fold being held out of harm's way the bladder is opened and the finger quickly inserted to find the stone. Its size being noted, the incision is enlarged to permit its removal by the forceps. The stone being removed, careful search is made to see if any bits remain which may have been broken off during removal. The bladder is thoroughly irrigated and a T-shaped drainage tube introduced and the wound packed with iodoform gauze. Sometimes the bladder wall is closed, using the interrupted Lembert suture. This should only be done in selected cases where primary union is expected, as urinary infiltration and septic infection are likely to occur. Many surgeons advocate the transverse incision (Trendelenberg's), as it affords an easier and freer opening into the bladder. The mutilation, however, is greater, shock more profound and great tendency to subsequent ventral hernia. It, however, gives greater room for manipulation.

An absorbent antiseptic dressing is placed outside of the tube and the patient kept on his side on an air cushion. This position favors drainage. The tube can be removed about the fifth day. Boracic acid solution is used to irrigate the bladder two or three times every twenty-four hours for the first few days. Sometimes it is advisable to close the upper third of the wound with sutures, and again splendid results have been obtained under conditions of improved technique by suturing the bladder and the greater part of the wound, leaving a small portion open for drainage.

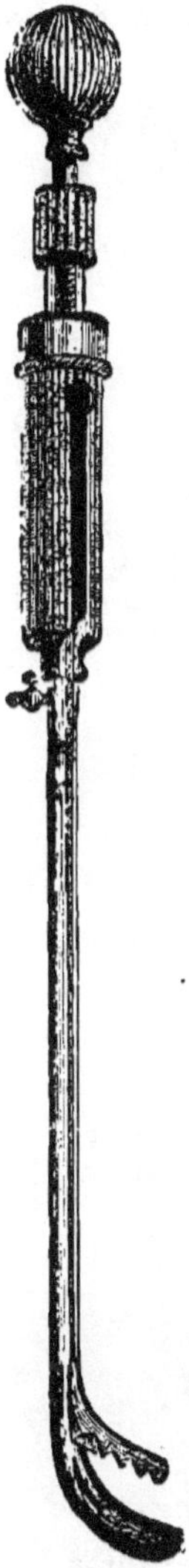

Litholapaxy.—This method consists of crushing the stone and removing the fragments at one sitting. Its introduction as a substitute for lithotrity by Bigelow, in 1878, marked an era in surgery of the bladder. The instruments proposed by the originator have stood the test of time in a highly satisfactory manner. It is an operation not entirely free from danger, the patient often being subjected to long and trying ordeals before the desired result is accomplished.

The principal instruments employed are lithotrites, large and small, an evacuator with tubes of several sizes, catheters and sounds. Bigelow's lithotrite (Fig. 35) is perhaps the best. Its construction admits of easy introduction into the bladder through the dilated urethra, and the mechanism of the jaws prevents impaction. When the stone is crushed the fragments are best removed by the aid of Bigelow's evacuator (Fig. 36), an instrument which perhaps has not been improved upon. The patient is to be prepared as for any other operation for stone, having partaken freely of some pure water, Poland, Clysmic or Bethesda, for a couple of days before the operation, and the same effort made to render the urine bland by the administration of some of the antiseptics previously

FIG. 35.

mentioned. The bladder should be washed out several times before the operation with a Boro-Salicylic solution and the rectum emptied. The patient, thoroughly anæsthetized, is placed upon his back upon a table and the urethra dilated to a No. 25 to No. 28 French scale. If necessary the meatus is cut to admit the instruments. Should strictures complicate they are to be divided or divulsed. Five or six ounces of fluid should be injected into the bladder and its outflow checked by tying a soft rubber tube about the penis. The lithotrite is now to be introduced. It is passed as a sound or catheter until the beak reaches the bulbous portion of the urethra. The lithotrite is now vertical, and the penis being drawn upward the obstruction offered by the triangular ligament is removed and the instrument slips into the membranous urethra. The handle is depressed gently between the thighs and the jaws glide along the prostatic urethra into the bladder. Should the beak of the instrument catch on the prostate the finger introduced into the rectum will guide it over the obstruction. Once in the bladder it is pushed to the posterior wall of the viscus. The male blade is now withdrawn until it reaches the vesical neck then gently pushed back. Should this manœuvre not be successful in catching the stone, the blades are opened again and turned on the side then closed, this movement being repeated on both sides. The degrees of rotation should be varied and the movements repeated. If there is a post-prostatic

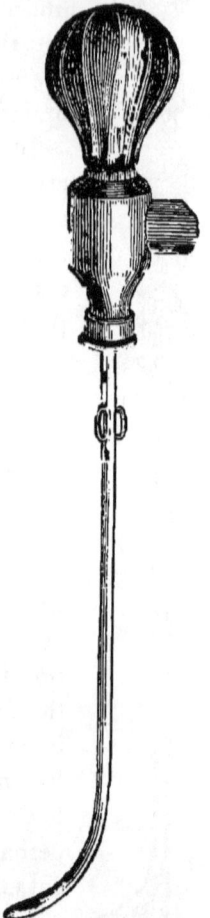

FIG. 36.

pouch the opened instrument should search there with the beak directed into it. This last movement often catches the mucous membrane. If the patient's hips are raised the stone will often fall out of the pouch, or it may be dislodged by the introduction of the finger into the rectum. Again in extreme cases this post-prostatic pouch may be entirely obliterated by the introduction of a rubber colpeurynter into the rectum as suggested by Buckston Browne.

With each new position of the lithotrite the male blade is pushed gently home. Should the stone be within its grasp the button is moved, the screw connected to hold the stone and the instrument rotated to the centre of the bladder. If the mucous membrane has been caught the operator becomes aware of the fact at this moment. If it seems to be free the screw is turned slowly and gently at first to secure the stone safely in the jaws of the instrument, then sufficient force is applied to produce fragmentation. If the calculus is very hard it often slips from the jaws of the instrument, particularly when it has not been caught in a favorable diameter. Again, if too hard, the screw cannot be turned. If soft the male blade advances evenly with each turn of the screw. After the stone is broken the fragments are picked up separately and crushed much in the same manner as was employed originally for the intact stone. With the small fragments it is not always necessary to put on the screw power, but they may be crushed by simply pushing the male blade home with the hand; this admits of greater rapidity in the disposal of the smaller fragments. When finally no more fragments can be found or when the patient's limit of endurance seems to have been reached by the length of the *séance* the jaws of the instrument are carried to the centre of the bladder, the male blade pushed in and out several times to remove any impaction, then screwed firmly into its fellow and the instrument carefully removed from the bladder. The evacuating tube of the lithotrite is now introduced in the shape and size depending upon the condition of the tract. Usually a size equal to 28 or 30 French is selected, and if possible the straight tube should be employed, as it is easily turned in the bladder and affords a straight direct route for the passage of the fragments. When introduced it is attached to the bulb, which is held in the right hand while the tube is steadied with the left. The distal end of the tube is depressed so that the proximal opening is not buried in the *detritus*. Compression of the bulb at first, according to Bigelow, should be slight and rapid. This produces a commotion in the bladder which sends the fragments rapidly through the fluid and they may be caught while in a state of momentary suspension. Sometimes the tube is blocked by a large fragment or a fold of mucous membrane covers the opening; either may be dislodged by an abrupt forcible compression of the bulb. When the bladder walls are so caught it is an evidence that the solution is low, but may be replenished by dropping the rubber evacuating tube into the Boro-Salicylic solution, closing the stop-cock to the bladder tube, thus filling the evacuator, then forcing it into the bladder. The last fragment is often difficult to find, or rather to remove, and it is often necessary to introduce a smaller lithotrite to crush it. When no more clicks can be heard or felt a sound is introduced and the cavity of the bladder carefully examined. A small tube, preferably a rubber catheter, is introduced and the bladder washed for the last time; the fluid is allowed to run along the urethra to wash out any *débris* that may have lodged there. The patient should be placed in bed and, if possible, allowed to urinate naturally. A milk diet with frequent libations of water, and Salol or Boracic acid by the mouth constitutes the after treatment. A large soft catheter may be introduced several days afterwards to remove tenacious mucus or blood clots which may have collected after the operation.

STONE IN THE FEMALE BLADDER.—Stone in

the bladder is not common among women, the large and easily dilatable urethra affording opportunity for small calculi to escape before their size is increased by further deposition of salts. The causes, symptoms and diagnosis are practically the same as in the case of males.

Treatment.—Dilatation of the urethra: This is to be accomplished with urethral or uterine sounds and then with the finger. When sufficient dilatation has been secured the stone, if small, may be removed with forceps or clasp. If too large to remove in this way sufficient dilatation is made to introduce a lithotrite and the stone is crushed. This is the method to choose in the majority of cases of stone in women. For evacuation a short tube of larger calibre should be employed. Vaginal or suprapubic lithotomy is to be employed when litholapaxy is impracticable. In the latter operation the patient is placed in Sims' position, a sound is introduced into the bladder and made prominent on the vesico-vaginal septum. This point is incised and the opening enlarged sufficiently to extract the stone. The wound should be kept open and if necessary the plan suggested by Emmet employed, that of stitching the vaginal and vesical mucous membranes together, and when the bladder has been sufficiently drained the opening is closed by the operation for vesico-vaginal fistula. As a rule the wound made in the ordinary manner if left to itself heals spontaneously.

CHAPTER XII.

PYELITIS.

Pyelitis is an inflammation of the pelvis and calices of the kidney.

Etiology.—It may attack one or both, affecting one side when the cause is not lower down than the ureter and is local in character. When both are affected it may result from constitutional disorders, diseases of the bladder, prostate gland or stricture of the urethra.

It is never idiopathic and is always secondary to some other diseased condition. It may be acute or chronic, calculous or tubercular.

Acute pyelitis may occur during infectious diseases, gonorrhœa, etc. It is of short duration and often passes unnoticed.

Chronic pyelitis is the result of obstruction to the urinary flow by strictures, enlarged prostate, chronic cystitis, pressure of tumors on, or a retained stone in the ureter, etc.

Calculous pyelitis is produced by the presence of calculi in the pelvis of the kidney. If these can be dissolved or dislodged the case can be cured, otherwise they will increase in size and the symptoms of pyelitis will become more distressing.

Tubercular pyelitis is dependent upon tubercular growths in the pelvis of the kidney.

Pathological Anatomy.—In acute pyelitis the mucous membrane is congested and hyperæmic, dotted here and there with minute ecchymotic spots and small areas denuded of epithelium. The whole surface is covered with pus and muco-pus. In diphtheritic pyelitis the exudation is plastic in character.

In the chronic form the membrane is thickened, of a

grayish-white or slate color, the walls dilated and sacculated, the veins prominent, the surface granulated and ulcerated, covered with pus, which may contain minute fragments of calculous formation. The pelvis may be distended with thick pus and phosphates, and the kidney tissue much atrophied, or the parenchyma may undergo complete atrophy, forming an abscess, which in some cases ruptures into the surrounding parts with or without accompanying adhesive inflammation.

Clinical History.—There will be pain referred to the lumbar region of one or both sides, with soreness and tenderness on deep pressure. The pain follows the direction of the ureter, and shoots into the perinæum and thigh and is accompanied by frequent, painful urination, this condition often leading to the diagnosis of cystitis, the pyelitis being overlooked.

Acute pyelitis may be ushered in by marked rigors, followed by a general catarrhal fever. In the gonorrhœal form fever is absent, the pain is slight, and in gonorrhœal cystitis this condition often passes unrecognized.

The urine is acid in reaction with a specific gravity of about 1030, containing blood, pus-corpuscles, mucus, tailed epithelium, etc. As the disease becomes more chronic the quantity of pus increases. It does not collect in masses, it is not ropy, but remains separated, giving a turbid appearance to the urine, but on standing it settles to the bottom of the vessel. As the disease progresses the epithelial cells gradually disappear from the urine, which always remains acid, differing from the alkaline urine of cystitis.

If the pelvis of the kidney becomes sacculated the urine will be ammoniacal, and sometimes the breath and perspiration will exhale the peculiar odor of ammonia. In these cases beware of urethral operations. The amount of albumen in the urine varies according to the quantity of pus and blood present. In pyelitis, when the ureter is free throughout its whole extent, pus will be constantly found in the urine, but if it is obstructed a tumor will be developed between the crest of the ilium and the last rib, giving a slight prominence to the affected side. When the obstruction is removed this tumor will disappear and large quantities of pus will be discharged with the urine.

The symptoms of pyelitis are always modified by the cause, whether of obstructive, tubercular or calculous origin. The tubercular form can be detected by the presence of the tubercular bacilli in the urine. The pyelitis resulting from the presence of calculi is more painful than the ordinary form, the pains in the region of the kidney and the quantity of pus and blood in the urine being increased by motion. Rest in the recumbent position for a few days causes the disappearance of the symptoms.

In chronic pyelitis there will be some fever, emaciation and weakness, often chill, fever and sweat (hectic), occurring at regular intervals, generally in the evening. This is especially true in conditions of pyo-nephrosis from occlusion of the ureter. When the pelvis of only one kidney is affected the kidney structure sometimes becomes involved and absorbed, resulting in the formation of an encysted collection of pus. The kidney of the opposite side undergoes compensatory hypertrophy.

The abscess may rupture and burrow into the surrounding tissue, opening either in the back, under Poupart's ligament, into the bladder, sometimes into the lungs and rarely the peritoneum. Incision should be made early in all cases where there is evidence of pus in the region of the kidney, as it will be less dangerous than if left to burrow. When it is opened or rupture occurs the discharge will soon cease, unless a calculus or foreign body remains in the pus cavity, when the discharge will persist and the wound remain open.

Treatment.—Direct attention to the cause and remove it. In the acute condition the appropriate remedy is usually the one indicated by the general condition. The use of drugs which may have produced irritation, as Turpentine, Copaiva, Sandal-wood, etc., must be discontinued. When the trouble results from calculi the administration of Hydrangea, Lycopodium, Silicea and Piperazine for the uric acid form, and Magnesium boro-citrate when from the phosphates and oxalates, has often caused the disappearance of the symptoms. If the calculi are not dissolved and Uva ursi, Mercurius corrosivus, Thuja, Cantharis, Cannabis sativa and Stigmata maidis fail to give relief, a nephrotomy must be performed if the condition of the patient permits it; if an abscess has formed and points an operation should be made at once. First withdraw some of the pus with the aspirating needle, then open freely and dress antiseptically. In this operation there is no danger of opening into the peritoneal cavity, as the kidney is outside and behind it.

GRAVEL.—This condition is the result of an excessive formation of solid matter and its condensation or deposit in the urine. The symptoms are caused by their passage through the urinary tract. These calculi, or gravel stones, irregular in shape, are always recognized by the microscope and often with the unaided eye. They are composed of urates, phosphates, oxalates, etc., and are the result of over-concentration of the urine from dyspepsia, ingestion of sweet wines, malted liquors, over-indulgence at the table with little exercise; also of sexual disorders, over-acid condition of the system from any cause, as in gout, rheumatism, etc.

Clinical History.—There is smarting and burning on micturition, with irritation and congestion of the urinary tract, pain and uneasiness, referred to the sacro-iliac region, shooting down the course of the ureter, together with irritation at the neck of the bladder, headache, flatulence, malaise, etc. If the condition is not soon rectified it may result in calculous pyelitis, or if the small stones pass into the bladder during an attack of renal colic they may be voided with the urine from the bladder or remain as nuclei for the formation of vesical calculi. An over-acid and concentrated urine alone will keep up a long train of symptoms and finally causes or terminates in pyelitis, cystitis, etc.

Treatment.—Strict dietary regulations must be observed.

Reduce the quantity of meat and increase the average amount of vegetables. Light meals must be the rule.

Prohibit champagne, sweet and new wines, malted and spirituous liquors. Sedentary habits must be abandoned and out-door exercise gradually adopted and continued. Frequent bathing, Turkish or Russian baths. Massage once or twice weekly and frequent rubbing with a rough bath towel or flesh brush are productive of much good. Sexual hygiene is important, especially in the young.

A pint of Piperazin water should be drank daily in divided doses; it is prepared as follows:

℞ Piperazin, ... grammes v.
Aqua Destil., ... ℥v.
M.

Sig. Tablespoonful to a pint of any mineral water.

Mineral and distilled water in large quantities should be advised and the alkaline flow of urine, which occurs usually about 10.30 A. M., if absent, should be re-established and maintained. When the alkaline waters do not produce the desired results administer 30 grains of Citrate of Potash, well diluted with water, at bed time and between meals.

The alkaline condition of the urine prevents the deposit of the solid matters in the urinary tract, while acidity facilitates it. Whenever the urine for any length of time remains acid for the entire day it indicates over-acidity and concentration. These conditions give rise to many, if not all, of the symptoms of gravel and neuralgia of the kidneys.

When the urine is acid the indicated remedy may be Lycopodium, Sepia, Magnesium boro-citrate, Quinia sulph. or Sarsaparilla, and when alkaline Phosphoric acid.

RENAL CALCULI.—These may be composed of urates, phosphates or oxalate of lime. When they attain a considerable size in the pelvis of the kidney they may cause symptoms of pyelitis or nephralgia. If the calculi are carried into the ureter they produce sudden and severe pain, which continues until they are discharged into the bladder.

RENAL COLIC.—This is caused by the passage of a renal calculus, a hydatid, or clot of blood or pus through the ureter. The pain varies greatly in severity and duration, according to the condition of the ureter and the size and shape of the foreign body.

Clinical History.—Renal colic may be moderate in severity, continuing only a few minutes, or it may be agonizing and last for hours or days; sometimes it is intermittent in character. It commences suddenly, although it may be preceded by some pain and uneasiness which is referred to the lumbar region of the affected side; it ends almost as suddenly when the stone or foreign body enters the bladder.

When the foreign body engages at the opening of the ureter in the pelvis of the kidney it causes pain which is referred to the affected side. If, on the other hand, it becomes disengaged and passes back into the pelvis of the kidney the pain will cease for the time being, to return when the foreign body re-enters the ureter.

If it is to pass, the pain, which usually commences suddenly, increases in violence, follows the course of the ureter and shoots down the inner side of the thigh to the end of the penis and into the scrotum, which is frequently retracted by the contraction of the cremaster muscle. The pain may radiate in various directions over the abdomen to the breast or up the back; it is paroxysmal, and so agonizing at times that it often, in nervous people, causes convulsions or syncope. As the attack increases in violence the patient rolls and twists from side to side and from one position to another in the endeavor to find relief. The face becomes pale, anxious, covered with perspiration, and the suffering is so great that he frequently screams and moans like a woman in labor. The pain continues between the paroxysms, but is less severe. There is an ineffectual desire to urinate, which is accompanied with burning, the urine being small in quantity and of dark color. When the pain is very severe there may be rectal tenesmus together with a small unsatisfactory stool. Vomiting is of frequent occurrence. Unless the pain continues for some time there is usually no rise in temperature nor change in the pulse. If the foreign body becomes impacted in the ureter the intense pain may gradually subside and become gnawing in character, being referred to the affected locality. This again may disappear if the ureter enlarges to allow the urine to pass along beside the foreign body, but when it entirely occludes the ureter it leads to hydro- or pyo-nephrosis.

After passing into the bladder the calculus is usually expelled with the flow of urine during the next few hours; it may have caused great pain when passing through the ureter, but, if the urethra is normal, it may be passed without notice or pain. In order to ascertain the character of the foreign body causing the colic the urine must be carefully examined at each urination until the obstructing body has been found.

The prognosis is always good unless impaction occurs, resulting in hydro- or pyo-nephrosis, etc. One attack predisposes to another. After the attack there is profuse micturition, but the urine may contain blood for some days from injury to the ureters.

Treatment.—Between the attacks the treatment is that recommended for gravel, together with the administration of Hydrangea, Lycopodium, Sepia, Magnesium borocitrate or Quinia sulph. During the attack hot baths (general or sitz), hot fomentations or a hot water bag over the affected parts. Alkaline waters in large quantities, Citrate of Potash in 20-grain doses well diluted, every three hours, and light beers have been recommended to increase the flow of urine and so force the obstructing body onward. Change of position and manipulation of the parts often give relief and dislodge the mass. The inhalation of Ether or Chloroform sometimes gives speedy relief. Suppositories of Opium and Belladonna are useful and act satisfactorily, but many physicians when called administer a hypodermic of Morphia ($\frac{1}{8}$ to $\frac{1}{2}$ grain combined with $\frac{1}{120}$ of a grain of Atropia), the dose being regulated according to the intensity of the pain and repeated as required. The patient usually quiets down, becomes easy or falls asleep to awake free from pain and possibly only a little soreness of the parts.

With some, however, the use of Morphia is followed by many unpleasant symptoms, especially so in the gouty. It may be the direct cause of bringing on an attack of gout which may be more painful than the colic itself. In these and many other cases satisfactory results have been obtained by the administration of Dioscorea, Berberis, Hydrangea or Coccus cacti; relief is not immediate, but they escape the attack of gout. The passage of a full-sized steel sound into the bladder has been recommended and used with satisfactory results; its action is probably reflex, causing the ureters to dilate and allow the urine behind to push the obstruction into the bladder.

CHAPTER XIII.

SPECIAL THERAPY FOR THE PROSTATE, BLADDER, URETERS AND PELVIS OF THE KIDNEY.

Aconite.—Acute prostatitis. Cystitis and retention of urine. Inflammation and congestion of the mucous membrane of the entire urinary tract. Painful micturition with great anxiety. Urine scanty, red and hot. Burning in the urethra after micturition. Retention of urine from sudden chilling of the surface. Tenesmus with burning at the neck of the bladder. Enuresis with thirst. Inflammation of the bladder and kidneys; region of kidneys sensitive to touch. Tenderness over the hypogastric region. Violent burning in the bladder with frequent straining; urine mixed with blood. Restlessness. Skin hot and dry. Hard, quick, full pulse.

Aloe Socotrina.—Incontinence of urine of the aged, with each act feels as if he must have a small stool. Bearing down sensation with enlarged prostate. Sensation of a plug between the sacrum and the coccyx.

Alumina.—High colored urine, which can only be passed when straining at stool.

Apis.—Urine dark-red and scanty. Inflammation of the bladder. Vesical tenesmus. Incontinence of the urine with great irritation of the parts. Burning and soreness when urinating.

Argentum Nitricum.—Hypertrophy of the prostate. Urine high colored, scanty and strong smelling. Inability to pass urine in a projecting stream. Incontinence of urine, especially in the aged.

Arnica.—Injuries of the prostate, bladder or ureters. Bloody urine from mechanical violence. Tenesmus. Frequent desire to urinate with involuntary urination. Retention. Involuntary micturition during the day or when moving. Urine brown, high colored, bloody, containing phosphates. Urine passed drop by drop, has to wait some time before the act can be commenced. Pressing pain in kidney and ureters after the passage of a calculus with bloody urine.

Arsenicum Album.—Atony of the bladder with retention. Difficult micturition. Burning pain, especially on beginning to urinate. Face pale, extremities cold, restlessness, fever. Bladder greatly over-distended. Involuntary micturition from paralysis of the bladder (overflow). Involuntary enuresis at night during sleep. Tenesmus. Strangury. Urine mixed with pus, turbid, greenish, foul smelling, slimy, dark brown sediment. Uræmic condition. Urinary fever. Fetid diarrhœa.

Aurum Met.—Retention of the urine. Tenesmus and frequent desire to urinate. Urine turbid, like buttermilk, with a thick sediment of mucus. Heat starting from the kidneys and extending to the bladder. Pain in the lumbar region, extending down the side. Pyelitis.

Belladonna.—Acute cystitis. Irritable bladder from hyperæsthesia. The region of the bladder is very sensitive to touch. Incontinence of urine. Enuresis at night with sudden starting up from sleep as if frightened. Spasm of the urethra. Retention of urine. Urine passed with difficulty, drop by drop, with tenesmus and constant desire. Urine sometimes bloody. Continual dribbling of urine. Urine scanty, red, turbid, dark, sometimes as yellow as gold. Sharp stitching pain in the perinæum, which comes suddenly and disappears as suddenly.

Benzoic Acid.—Cystitis. Prostatitis. Pyelitis. Frequent urination. Irritable bladder. Nocturnal enuresis of children. Enlarged prostate. Urine offensive, brown, containing pus and mucus. Urine changeable in odor, usually very disagreeable and offensive, cloudy, alkaline in reaction, containing phosphates and carbonates in large quantities. Urine sometimes thick and bloody. Weariness in the inguinal regions. The patient pale and anæmic. Frequent desire to urinate with tenesmus. Specific gravity of urine increased from increase of uric acid. Urine offensive, smelling like horse urine.

Berberis Vulgaris.—Renal colic. Gravel. Pyelitis. Cystitis. Vesical irritability. Burning, cutting and sticking pain in the urethra. Frequent micturition with burning before and during the act, especially in the female. Violent stitching, tearing, burning pain in the region of the kidney, extending forward along the course of the ureters into the bladder, to the posterior part of the pelvis and thighs; worse when stooping, lying or sitting, relieved by standing. Stitches from the kidney to the bladder with frequent desire to urinate. Drawing, tensive, tearing pains in the lumbar region. Violent stitches in the bladder with frequent urination. Cutting, constrictive pain in bladder, whether full or empty. Desire to urinate with burning in urethra. Burning in the urethra after urination. Motion aggravates the urinary troubles; pain in the loins and hips generally accompanying the symptoms. Urine yellow, red with reddish and bran-like sediment. Blood-red urine. Greenish urine, pale yellow with slight, transparent, gelatinous sediment which does not deposit; or a turbid, flocculent, clay-colored, copious mucous sediment, mixed with white or whitish-gray, and later a reddish, mealy sediment. Pain in the testicles.

Calcarea Carb.—Involuntary discharge of urine when walking. Frequent micturition at night. Nocturnal enuresis, urine clear and sour smelling. Trickling of urine after urination. Offensive, dark urine, containing thick mucus and depositing a white sediment like flour.

Camphor.—Tenesmus of the neck of the bladder. Strangury. Retention of urine. Micturition frequent, difficult and painful, with dribbling of urine or with a thin stream as if the urethra were contracted. Frequent ineffectual urging to urinate. When urinating pressure in the region of the bladder and burning in the urethra. Urine scanty, red and thick or yellowish-green, turbid and offensive. Retention of urine.

Cannabis Indica.—Inflammation of the bladder with burning, scalding and stinging before, during and after urination. After urination much straining and strangury. Dribbling of urine after micturition. Copious discharge of clear white or thick red urine with burning.

Cantharis.—Acute cystitis. Retention of urine. Strangury. Gravel, especially in children. Congestive pyelitis. Constant and ineffectual urging to urinate. Cystitis, generally of gonorrhœal origin. Spasmodic pain in the bladder, with urgent desire to urinate. Intense burning in the bladder. Micturition painful, drop by drop with a feeling as though melted lead were passing down the urethra with violent straining, which increases the pain. Urine at first clear, but afterwards turbid, scanty or of blood only. Thirst, but drinking always increases the pains in the bladder. Burning, stinging and tearing in the region of the kidneys. Violent pressing pain in lumbar region, extending to the bladder. The cystitis calling for Cantharis is of a high inflammatory grade with hæmaturia; it may be accompanied by a chill, fever, etc. The specific gravity of the urine is always high and it is always acid, containing large quantities of urates. In the gravel of children the pains extend down the penis with a constant inclination to pull at the organ.

Carbo Veg.—Chronic cystitis of the aged. Pressing pain in the bladder. Urine has a strong odor, dark-colored, as if mixed with blood, and deposits a sediment.

Causticum.—Incontinence of urine, from want of power in the vesical sphincter. Paralysis of the bladder after labor, with retention of urine. Involuntary discharge of urine when coughing, during the first sleep at night, and from the least over-exertion or excitement. Pulsating pain in the perinæum. Pain in the bladder after a few drops of urine have been passed. Urging to urinate, but must wait a long time before he commences the act, which may afterwards be involuntary. Urine light colored, with flocculent sediment. Lithiates.

Chimaphila Umbellata.—Chronic cystitis. Vesical tenesmus, the urine containing large quantities of ropy mucus. Scanty urine. Inability to pass the urine without standing with the feet widely separated. Acute inflammation of the prostate, with a feeling as of a ball in the perinæum. Desire to urinate, with great burning and smarting, which is not relieved by micturition. This drug is very frequently indicated in both acute and chronic inflammation of the bladder; the urine is high colored, with a bloody, greenish or reddish sediment, but has particularly large quantities of thick, ropy, slimy, fetid mucus, with much muco-purulent deposit.

Chininum Sulph.—Gravel. Urine is scanty, acid, turbid, of strong odor, and flows slowly, with a sediment of yellowish-red crystals, or clear, containing four-sided prisms, the pointed ends being enveloped in mucus. Urine turbid, alkaline, chocolate-colored, with phosphates increased. Cramping and neuralgic pains in the region of the kidneys. Sediments yellowish-white, mealy, of strong odor, brick-dust, slimy flakes, with large numbers of transparent, colorless and orange-colored crystals, star-like, rhomboidal and flat crystals, mostly phosphates.

Coccus Cacti.—Renal colic. Chronic cystitis. Drawing, lancinating pain in the lumbar region, extending along the course of the ureters. Cutting and heaviness in the bladder and constant urging to urinate, relieved by micturition. Frequent ineffectual attempts to urinate at night; has to wait a long time before he can succeed. Retention of urine until there is intense pain, when a small amount is passed slowly, with much suffering. Pain and soreness in the region of the bladder. Hæmaturia.

Urine contains large deposits of urates and Uric acid, and is thick, hot, acrid and burning.

Colchicum.—Frequent desire to urinate; urine is dark and scanty, depositing a whitish sediment.

Colocynthis.—Frequent discharge of a small quantity of urine with tenesmus, and followed by burning in the urethra Urine viscid, like thin glue, which thickens on standing and is fetid. Urine turbid, with copious deposit of hard, reddish crystals. Uric acid. Chlorides diminished.

Conium.—Chronic prostatitis. Much difficulty in voiding the urine; it flows and stops, then starts and flows again at each emission. Frequent urination during the night. Pressure on the bladder, the urine cannot be retained. Pressing pain and stitches at the neck of the bladder, worse from motion, better on sitting. Urine thick, white and turbid.

Copaiva.—Acute cystitis, especially in the course of a gonorrhœa. Constant desire to urinate. Intense inflammation of the bladder, especially at the neck. Burning and a sensation of dryness in the region of the prostate gland and neck of bladder, urine passed in drops, with great pain and straining. Urine foaming, greenish, turbid, bloody, smelling like violets. Irritability of the neck of bladder and urethra in old women.

Cubeba.—Cystitis. Tenesmus, with smarting on the passage of the urine, which may be foamy and contain ropy mucus.

Digitalis.—Throbbing pain in the region of the neck of the bladder during micturition. Increased desire to urinate after a few drops have been passed, causing great distress and associated with tenesmus of the rectum. Ineffectual efforts to urinate, with the discharge of a few drops of urine and a continual fullness after urinating. Urine is dark brown, hot and burning when passed. Excessive quantity of urine. The urine is retained more easily in the recumbent position.

Dulcamara.—Cystitis, especially when caused by exposure to cold or damp, and where the disease tends to become chronic, or in chronic cases which are aggravated by a change to damp, cold weather. Urine turbid, white, or fetid. Painful, frequent urination. Retention. Involuntary discharge of urine, from atony of the bladder. Thickening of the muscular coats in chronic cystitis.

Dioscorea.—Renal colic; has acted very well and promptly.

Equisetum.—Nocturnal enuresis. Incontinence of urine in the aged, especially in women. Pain in the bladder not relieved by urinating. Pain as from distention. Constant desire to urinate, which micturition does not relieve. Tenderness over the bladder. Frequent desire to urinate, but only a small quantity is passed. Weakness of the bladder, dribbling of urine, and pain as from over-distention. Urine scanty, high-colored, bloody, albuminous, showing great excess of mucus on standing.

Erigeron.—Catarrh of the bladder, with much pain. Children cry when urinating, from the pain. Urine profuse, bloody, of strong odor. Stone in the bladder.

Eucalyptus.—Chronic catarrh of the bladder and genito-urinary tract. The urine smells like violets.

Gelsemium.—Frequent desire to evacuate the bladder with discharge of copious, limpid urine relieving the dullness and heaviness of the head. Constant dribbling of urine from muscular weakness. Bladder distended with urine; retention and overflow. Enuresis at night. Dysuria and spasmodic retention of urine from cold, etc. Feeling on urinating as if some of the urine remained behind, with a small intermittent stream. Post-diphtheritic paralysis of the sphincter.

Graphites.—Frequent micturition, especially at night.

Urine sour-smelling, depositing a thick sediment with pain in sacrum on urinating.

Hepar Sulphuris.—Pyelitis. Micturition slow, has to wait some time for the urine to flow, when it does so slowly; it may drop straight down from the end of the penis. The patient is never able to finish, he always feels as if some was left in the bladder. Urine is dark-red, hot, and becomes thick, turbid and deposits a white sediment on standing.

Hydrangea is a valuable and important remedy for gravel and for preventing the return of renal colic. In a large number of cases where it was given for some months without special dieting there has been no return of the trouble. It causes the excess of urates and white amorphous salts to disappear from the urine. It should be given in seven drop doses of the fluid extract in a little water, four times daily.

Hydrastis.—Catarrhal inflammation of the bladder with thick, ropy mucus in the urine.

Hyoscyamus.—Retention of urine, bladder distended. Involuntary discharge of urine. Frequent micturition. Prolapsus of the bladder. Difficult micturition, must strain from pressure. Urine turbid, depositing mucus or a purulent sediment. Difficult micturition, inflammation not far advanced; in cases where the trouble is more spasmodic than inflammatory.

Ignatia.—Sensation of scraping and smarting in the neck of the bladder. Sudden, irresistible desire to urinate, especially when walking. Frequent discharge of watery urine. Pressure to urinate from drinking coffee. Urine lemon-colored with white sediment.

Iodium.—Induration and atrophy of the prostate. Inflammation of the prostate in scrofulous and tubercular subjects.

Kali Bichromicum.—Stitching pain in the prostate gland on walking. Painful drawing from perinæum to urethra. After micturition sensation as if a drop remained behind. Escape of prostatic fluid at stool.

Kreosotum.—Urine has an offensive smell and is of deep red color, with reddish sediment.

Lachesis.—Urging and inability to urinate with pressure and dull pain in the bladder. Sensation of a ball rolling in the bladder on turning in bed. Urine profuse, foaming and offensive, varying from a coffee color to black and discharge of a bad looking mucus with the urine.

Lycopodium.—Chronic cystitis. Gravel. Prostatitis. Dull pressing pains and stitches in the bladder. Stitches in the neck of the bladder and anus at the same time. Pressing pain in perinæum during and after micturition. Urging to urinate, must wait some time before he can pass it. Frequent desire to urinate with scanty flow. Terrific pain in the back previous to each urination, relieved as soon as the flow begins. Smarting and burning when urinating. Drawing, cutting pain through to the abdomen. Pain in the kidney and bladder with frequent urination. Renal colic from the passage of small calculi; pain is burning and cutting in character. Calculus with bloody urine. Urine profuse, dark, bloody, with much red, sandy sediment. Greasy pedicle in urine. Red sand on child's diaper. Before micturition the child screams with pain. Urine scanty and red. Copious, red, sandy deposits. Urine turbid, milky, with a thick purulent sediment and offensive odor. Aching pain in rectum.

Mercurius.—Prostatitis. Cystitis. Feeling of great pressure and heat in the perinæum. Heaviness and aching in the gland, which is swollen and hard. The urinary stream is exceedingly small, passed drop by drop, with a whitish sediment. Soreness to touch in the region of the bladder. Urgent desire to urinate, the urine may contain mucus, pus or blood. Gonorrhœal cystitis. Urine is turbid and fetid.

Nitric Acid.—Cystitis. Pyelitis. Contractive pain from

the kidney towards the bladder. Pain in the lumbar region. Burning pain in the bladder. Urging after micturition with shuddering along the spine. Burning pain in the urethra and cutting pain in the abdomen on urinating. Incontinence in old, broken-down men. Enuresis. Urine is offensive and contains pus and mucus. Urine ammoniacal; smells like horse urine, with white sediment. Bloody urine. Urine is cold when passed.

Nux Vomica.—Irritable and gouty bladder. Prostatitis. Spasmodic retention of urine. Frequent desire to urinate, but little is passed at a time and is accompanied by much burning. Painful and ineffectual efforts to urinate. Burning and tearing pain in the neck of the bladder on urinating. Violent straining when urinating. Paralysis of the bladder; the urine flows drop by drop as it is formed. Urine pale, containing thick, white mucus or purulent matter. Dark urine, depositing a red brick-dust sediment. Bloody urine. Strangury.

Ocimum Can.—Renal colic. Gravel. Cramping pain in the kidney, especially the right. Renal colic with micturition every fifteen minutes, the pain causing the patient to wring his hands, moaning and crying all the time. Urine red with brick-dust sediment and blood. Saffron-colored urine. Turbid urine, depositing a white albuminous sediment. Burning during micturition. Pain in ureters and deposit in urine of a large quantity of red sand.

Opium.—Atony of the bladder. Vesical calculi. Retention of the urine, and the sensibility is so blunted that the urine passes unnoticed. The urine is only passed after much effort. Lemon-colored urine with more or less sediment.

Pareira Brava.—Cystitis. Violent urging and straining to urinate, pain extends into the glans penis and down the thighs, even into the feet. Strangury. The pain is so agonizing that the patient can only urinate when on his knees with the head pressed against the floor. Paroxysms occur after midnight. Great burning on urinating. The urine is ammoniacal, containing thick, white viscid mucus.

Petroleum.—Involuntary discharge of reddish-brown, fetid urine.

Phosphoric Acid.—Cramps in the region of the kidney. Abnormal alkaline urine. The urine looks like milk and decomposes quickly.

Phosphorus.—White flocculent sediment in the urine. Acrid, offensive urine. Bloody urine. Thick, turbid, scanty urine. Bloody urine with pain in region of the kidneys.

Plumbum.—Paralysis of the bladder from spinal disease. Atony of the bladder. Tenesmus and difficult urination. Urine dark-colored and passed drop by drop. Urine scanty. The patient is unable to urinate because he lacks sensation to make the will act on the bladder.

Pulsatilla.—Prostatitis. Cystitis. Prostate gland swollen and inflamed. Pain at the neck of the bladder, with an intermitting stream of urine and spasmodic, contracting pains at the end of urination. Frequent desire to urinate. Spasmodic pain at the neck of the bladder extending to the pelvis and thighs. Frequent and almost ineffectual urging to urinate. Involuntary urination at night in bed. Constant pressure in the bladder with frequent desire to urinate. The urine is discharged while walking or standing. Urine bloody; reddish; mucous; jelly-like, slimy and sticks to the chamber. Brick-dust sediment.

Populus Trem.—Catarrh of the bladder. Severe tenesmus of old people on voiding urine which contains large quantities of mucus and pus. Pressure and aching in the pelvis. Enlarged prostate.

Prunus Spinosa.—Irritability of neck of bladder. Tenesmus. Must urinate every fifteen minutes. Burning pain in sphincter. Burning pain and ineffectual urging to urinate. Relief on passing the urine, but there remains a sticking pain in the glans penis which causes a spasm of the urethra and rectum. Strangury. Urine scanty and brown.

Rhus Aromatica.—Involuntary micturition day or night. Burning pain on urinating. Catarrh of the bladder. Prostatic enlargements.

Rhus Tox.—Incontinence of urine during rest. Snow-white sediment in the urine. Vesical tenesmus. Discharge of blood-red urine in drops. Retention of urine from getting wet. Urine is passed slowly. Dark urine soon becoming turbid.

Ruta Graveolens.—Pressure at the neck of the bladder after urinating as though it was still full. Involuntary micturition at night in bed, and even during the day on motion. Frequent micturition at night.

Sandal Wood.—Prostatitis. Cystitis. Deep pain and uneasiness in the perinæum. Urinary stream small and passed with difficulty Sensation of a ball at the neck of the bladder, increased on standing, relieved by exercise. Desire to change position.

Sabina.—Retention of urine. Diminished flow with tenesmus. Frequent urination with profuse flow of urine. Bloody urine.

Sabal Serrulata.—Prostatitis. Cystitis. Incontinence of urine. Prostate gland is enlarged and inflamed. Thin stream, flow intermittent, has to wait for the first drop. Tenesmus, frequent urging. Micturition unsatisfactory, passes but a few drops at a time. Intense straining when urinating. Crying and screaming when urinating. Incontinence of urine during the day from lifting, straining or laughing. Acute inflammation of prostate in old cases. Prostate swollen, hot and painful.

Sarsaparilla.—Gravel. Cystitis. Pain in the lumbar region going forward. Abdomen distended. Severe tenesmus; passes gravel and small calculi. Painful constriction of the bladder. Micturition frequent and ineffectual, ending by passing some blood; chills run from the bladder to the back. Gravel passes after urinating; has to get up in the night frequently to urinate. Retention of urine. Urine copious; clear; white; scanty and slimy; clay-colored and scanty. Sand in the urine or on the diaper. Child screams before and during micturition. The urine contains pus, blood and mucus. Fiery red, turbid urine with long flakes. Urine excoriating.

Selenium.—Prostatitis. Watery, sticky discharge just before stool and soon afterwards, or a drop of prostatic fluid dribbles away with an uncomfortable sensation while sitting. The patient is unable to urinate; has to wait for some time, followed by involuntary dribbling. Dark-red, scanty urine, with more or less sandy sediment.

Sepia.—Chronic cystitis. Gravel. Prostatitis. Pyelitis. The lower part of the abdomen feels distended, with tension and soreness. Frequent painful and ineffectual urging to urinate, until long effort and waiting have about tired out the sufferer. Desire to urinate, with bearing down in the pelvis. Burning and cutting when urinating. Nocturnal enuresis during the first sleep or on going to sleep. Urine dark, turbid, and mixed with pus; thick, slimy, turbid and offensive, depositing a pasty sediment. Chill and heat in the head during and after micturition. Pulsation in the small of the back. Sprained pain over the hips. Pain in the lumbar region. Deep-seated pressive pain and tension in the lumbar region. The discharge of mucus in the urine does not take place every time the the urine is passed, but occurs periodically. Fetid urine, with reddish, clay-colored sediment adhering to the chamber. The urine is so offensive that it must be removed at once.

Stigmata Maidis.—Renal colic. Gravel. Acute and chronic cystitis. Vesical tenesmus and irritation. Pyelitis. Retention of urine.

Staphisagria.—Prostatitis. Frequent desire to urinate

the urine is passed in a small stream or only in drops of dark urine with much urging. Burning at the neck of the bladder with urging, as if the bladder was not empty. Profuse, pale, watery urine, with much urging.

Sulphur.—Prostatitis. Cystitis. Pyelitis. Constant urging to urinate day and night, in a thin stream or drop by drop; the urine is high-colored and turbid, of penetrating odor, with thick deposit, which sticks to the chamber. Retention of urine. Urinates frequently, with a feeling of obstruction at the neck of the bladder and a sense of pressure and distention. Bruised sensation in small of back after micturition. The pains continue in the urethra until the urging to urinate returns. Increased secretion of urine. Frequent urination at night. The desire comes suddenly, is imperative, and if not gratified at once micturition becomes involuntary. The urine is clear, high-colored, turbid and excoriating.

Terebinth.—Strangury. Tenesmus of the bladder. Cystitis. Congestion of the urinary organs. Scanty, bright-colored, or bloody urine. Pressure in the bladder, extending to the kidneys, disappearing on walking. Burning and drawing in right kidney, extending to hip. Gonorrhœal pyelitis. Burning in the bladder, with violent dragging, cutting and burning pain. Urine scanty, bloody; black like coffee, turbid, with thick, dark sediment.

Thuja.—Prostatitis. Cystitis. Stitches from the rectum to the bladder and from the bladder to the urethra. Incontinence of urine, from paralysis of the sphincter. Frequent urging to urinate; the stream is often interrupted. Frequent micturition during the night. Discharge of a few drops of urine after urinating, with burning, stitching and itching in the urethra. The urine is clear when passed, but becomes cloudy on standing. Urine red, with brick-dust sediment.

Uva Ursi.—Pyelitis. Frequent desire to urinate. A small quantity of urine is passed with burning and followed by cutting at the neck of the bladder and great straining. The urine is slimy, yellow, purulent and bloody. Painfulness and soreness in the region of the kidney. Uneasy feeling in the left thigh and frequent desire to urinate; the stream is small with considerable effort to empty the bladder, which is done slowly. Pain and soreness in the left groin. Heavy pain in the lumbar region and uneasiness in the bladder. The urine is red, scanty, high-colored and acid.

CHAPTER XIV.

DISEASES OF THE SCROTUM AND TESTICLES.

PHTHEIRIASIS PUBIS.—This is commonly known as crabs. It is a pruriginous affection of the hairy parts of the genitals, especially the mons veneris, caused by the presence of parasites. It may invade all the hairy parts of the body except the scalp.

When a suspicious itching occurs on the genitals an examination should at once be made. The parasites multiply rapidly and their ova, which are attached to the hairs, can be seen with the unaided eye, and the parasite itself is firmly attached to the skin, from which it draws its sustenance. The parasites and their ova are conveyed from one person to another during coitus, by means of the clothing and even by the toilet. They cause intense biting and itching of the parts and some papular eruption.

Treatment.—The most satisfactory and rapid method will be to remove the hair, which, however, is not always necessary, and dust the parts with Calomel, or apply 10 grains of Mercurial ointment to the parts on retiring, being careful to protect the scrotum, and removing it the following morning with soap and hot water. It may be necessary to repeat the treatment. Ammoniated mercury ointment acts equally well, and its application is not so objectionable. A solution of Bi-chloride of Mercury 1 to 1000 applied to the parts every second day is very efficacious, but it should be continued for two weeks. The tincture of Delphinium staphisagria or Kerosene oil can also be used with satisfactory results.

CUTANEOUS DISEASES OF THE SCROTUM are very numerous and can generally be treated in the same manner as when the disease occurs elsewhere.

ERYTHEMATOUS INTERTRIGO.—This condition occurs in those who are fleshy and perspire freely. It can easily be relieved by washing the parts with a Carbolic acid solution (1–200), drying carefully and dusting with Oleate of Zinc, the parts being kept separated until healed by means of a suspensory bandage, the use of which should be continued for some time.

PRURIGO.—This is a very troublesome condition; it can be relieved by bathing the parts two or three times daily with a solution of Carbolic acid (1 to 200) together with change of air, general hygiene and the exhibition of the proper remedies, which are Muriatic acid, Nitric acid, Staphisagria, Antimonium crud., Aurum, Graphites, Rhus tox., Natrum sulph., Nux vomica, etc.

ELEPHANTIASIS SCROTI.—This is a hypertrophic overgrowth of the scrotum, rare in this country. The colored races are especially liable to the disease. It is ushered in by a local inflammatory condition, which subsides, leaving behind an enlargement of the parts. These attacks are repeated until the parts attain an enormous size; in one case the growth weighed 165 pounds.

Treatment.—Surgical.

HYPERTROPHY OF THE TESTICLE.—This may occur when only one has been developed or removed at an early age; when following the law of compensation the remaining testicle increases in size and does duty satisfactorily for both.

ATROPHY OF THE TESTICLE may occur as the result of orchitis, old age or wasting diseases.

A CRYPTORCHID is a male without testicles in the scrotum either from non-development or from retention in their descent into the scrotum. The cryptorchid possesses the power of performing the sexual act and may be sterile. This can only be decided by a microscopical examination of the seminal discharge.

A MONORCHID is a male with only one testicle in the scrotum the other having been retained in its descent.*

HYDROCELE.—This is an accumulation of serous or sero-fibrinous fluid within the tunica vaginalis, in a cyst connected with the testes or in some part of the spermatic cord.

Hydrocele may be acute or chronic, congenital, acquired, encysted or diffuse.

ACUTE HYDROCELE accompanies all inflammatory conditions of the testes or epididymis, and sometimes specific and tubercular orchitis. It is a simple inflammatory exudation, sero-plastic in character. As the primary disease disappears the fluid exudate is generally absorbed, but the plastic material may cause adhesion and obliteration of the sac. If the inflammation is severe suppuration may occur.

Treatment.—Rest and treatment as indicated for the originating cause. If the fluid distention is persistent Apis, Cantharis or Helleborus may cause absorption.

CHRONIC HYDROCELE is an effusion into the tunica vaginalis of an albuminous fluid, light amber or straw-colored, though it may be red, brown, chocolate or black from the admixture of blood. It varies in consistency from a thin liquid to a jelly-like substance containing cholesterine plates, epithelium, fatty particles, and sometimes spermatozoa and pus corpuscles.

---

*The testicles usually appear in the scrotal sac before birth, but they have been known to descend as late as the thirtieth year.

Etiology.—It may be caused by anything which disturbs the balance between secretion and absorption within the tunica vaginalis. Sometimes the cause cannot be discovered, but it is usually due to excessive secretion brought about by some mechanical irritation, as horseback riding, tight trousers, etc. It also occurs as a sympathetic affection in diseases of the bladder, urethra, cord and testes. It is more prevalent in warm than in cold climates.

Clinical History.—The amount of effusion varies greatly, from a few drachms to many ounces. The fluid accumulates slowly, without pain, and with so little inconvenience that it may not be noticed until the part has attained a considerable |size, though a dragging sensation in one or both sides of the scrotal sac is occasionally noticed. When the fluid accumulates rapidly the pain is intense, the presence of which indicates a high degree of inflammation, suppuration, or disease of the testes.

The swelling appears first at the most dependent portion of the scrotum which gradually increases, becoming pear-shaped, but if very large it may be spherical. The spermatic cord can easily be made out above the swelling. If the tunica vaginalis is not attached low down the upper part of the hydrocele may be elongated and extend upwards towards the ring. If old adhesions exist in the tunica vaginalis the swelling will be irregular.

Hydroceles are tense and cannot be compressed and are light in weight compared to their size; they are not sensitive to touch, thus differentiating from diseases of the testes.

The testicle is usually found in the posterior part of this fluid, a little below the centre. This point must be remembered, to avoid injuring the testicle when using the aspirating needle or trocar, which should be introduced in front and a little above the centre of the hydrocele. Sometimes the testicle is situated in front and below the centre, often being more or less displaced, but its location can be ascertained by a little manipulation, the presence of the organ being recognized by the sickening feeling which comes over the patient when it is squeezed. The diagnosis may be confirmed by the test of translucency if the walls of the tunica vaginalis have not been thickened by the deposit of plastic material or cartilaginous and calcified plates, sometimes formed in old cases of hydrocele. This test is a most satisfactory one when the effusion has been slow and the walls are thin and white, the fluid clear, free from blood, pus or other admixtures. The room must be darkened and a reflected light or candle placed in front of the suspected swelling, the surgeon standing behind and either shading the eye with the hand or looking through a short tube, the end of which is placed against the posterior wall of the swollen scrotum. If it is a hydrocele the whole mass will look clear and translucent, except where it is darkened by the outline of the testicle, thus verifying the diagnosis made by pressure. If the walls are much thickened or the cavity is filled with opaque fluid the aspirator must be relied upon to clear up the diagnosis.

The cutaneous layer of the scrotum is drawn somewhat tightly over the swollen tunica vaginalis. It is usually free from redness, heat and inflammation. The smooth, tense feel of hydrocele differentiates it from cancerous, tubercular or cystic growths. Fluctuation is easily demonstrated, but cough impulse is never present. The disease is progressive, and the quantity of fluid may become enormous, causing great inconvenience.

Surgical treatment may be palliative or radical. In infants hydrocele has been known to disappear after painting the scrotum with a weak solution of the tincture of Iodine or Collodion. The usual palliative treatment, however, is evacuation of the contents of the sac with a trocar or aspirator, which is performed as follows: The scrotum is washed with a Bichloride of Mercury solution, 1 to 1000.

the tumor is then held firmly in the left and the instrument in the right hand; the needle is then plunged obliquely upwards and backwards from the middle and front of the hydrocele and the fluid contents escape through it. Sometimes the sac does not refill, a reactive or adhesive inflammation setting in, especially in recent cases and in the aged, which closes the tunica vaginalis; usually, however, the fluid returns in a few weeks or months.

The radical treatment consists in not only the removal of the fluid, but also in the immediate introduction into the cavity of either Tincture of Iodine or Carbolic acid.

From one to eight drachms of the Tincture of Iodine have been successfully injected, but 30 to 60 minims are more frequently required. The Iodine causes great pain and swelling of the parts, refilling of the sac, fluctuation, etc., necessitating rest in bed for a few days and possibly the use of hot fomentations to the parts, together with the administration of anodynes, but the results are universally satisfactory. For some special reason a weaker solution is sometimes used. The Tincture of Iodine for the operation may be made with one part of Iodine crystals to ten parts of 95 per cent. alcohol; this is allowed to stand uncorked for a few days, when it will be ready for use. Of late years Carbolic acid has been frequently substituted for the Iodine; it has the advantage of being painless, and the inflammatory reaction from the injection takes place within twenty-four hours, and the patient is not detained from business more than a day, and sometimes not at all, the results being equally satisfactory. Thirty to one hundred minims of liquefied Carbolic acid (Carbolic acid crystals eight parts, Glycerine one part) are used. Sloughing never occurs after this injection, unless more that thirty minims have have used.

After either Carbolic acid or Iodine injections into the sac a certain amount of manipulation must be made to bring the injected fluid in contact with all the parts to insure complete adhesive inflammation. Others prefer to irrigate the tunica vaginalis, after withdrawing the fluid, with a three or four per cent. solution of Carbolic acid; this stops the excessive secretion of the serous coat, but does not set up an adhesive inflammation.

Injections of Carbolic acid or Iodine are contra-indicated if the withdrawn fluid contains blood or pus, or when the walls are thickened or calcareous.

Whether Iodine or Carbolic acid is used it is advisable for the patient to remain in bed for a day or two after the operation and wear a suspensory bandage for a few weeks. Setons have been used but are now obsolete. Electricity has cured some cases and Spongia, Pulsatilla, Rhododendron, Aurum, Graphites, Iodum, and Kali iod. have their recorded cures without surgical treatment.

CONGENITAL HYDROCELE.—This condition is most frequently met with in childhood and occasionally in adults. It is the result of imperfect obliteration of the communication between the peritoneum and its prolongation, known as the tunica vaginalis. Any fluid accumulating in the peritoneum flows easily into the sac, giving rise to symptoms which might be mistaken for hernia with which it is sometimes associated. This communication, however, is usually so small that only fluids can escape through it, the intestines and omentum remaining in the peritoneal cavity.

Congenital hydrocele appears or is noticed soon after birth; it has no well-defined upper border and is continuous with the inguinal canal. It can be readily reduced or made to return slowly into the peritoneal cavity by placing the patient in the dorsal position and elevating the scrotum, but it does not give the gurgling sound which is heard on reducing a hernia. On assuming the upright position the fluid quickly returns, cough impulse is present and the tumor gives flatness on percussion. When the sac is distended with fluid the testicle cannot be easily located, but when the contents have been emptied into the peritoneum the testicle will be found in its proper position.

Treatment.—A truss properly applied and remedies as indicated by the general condition. Operations are contraindicated.

ENCYSTED HYDROCELE.—This is an encysted accumulation, distinct from the tunica vaginalis, of a serous, opaque, limpid, milky fluid, usually containing spermatozoa. When occurring with chronic hydrocele it may remain undiscovered until operation, although attaining a large size. It usually begins in the head of the epididymis and grows slowly, accompanied by a slight pain which may have escaped notice. It is heart-shaped with the testicle below it. The patients are usually hypochondriacal.

Treatment is that advised for *chronic hydrocele*.

HYDROCELE OF THE CORD.—This may be diffuse or encysted.

DIFFUSE HYDROCELE of the cord is simply an œdema of or an effusion into the areolar tissue of a yellowish, limpid, albuminous fluid. It appears as a smooth rounded tumor, elongated, somewhat distended below, but it does not communicate with the tunica vaginalis. It is caused by some obstruction to the return circulation from the testicle and is of rare occurrence. It may occur spontaneously or develop after the application of some local irritant, as Iodine, etc.

Treatment.—Try the indicated remedy before operation.

ENCYSTED HYDROCELE OF THE CORD.—This condition does not often occur; it is recognized by the presence of one or more rounded and elongated swellings on the spermatic cord, situated anywhere between the internal opening of the inguinal canal and the testis. The elongations are in the direction of the cord and when large may be a little pyriform in shape; they vary in size from a millet seed to an egg and contain a straw-colored albuminous fluid. They are painless unless irritated. When located in the inguinal canal they are sometimes mistaken for incomplete hernia, and much pain and inconvenience has been caused by the consequent treatment.

Treatment.—If single, that advised for chronic hydrocele. When multiple, incision followed by antiseptic dressings gives the best results.

Remedies in hydrocele.—Arsenicum will be beneficial in old cases with weakness and debility. Dr. Richard Hughes reports a cure with Aurum. Calcarea carb. is indicated for scrofulous cases with general Calcarea symptoms, especially in childhood. China is sometimes useful. Conium when traced to mechanical injury. Dulcamara when caused from cold. Graphites if subject to eruptions, constipation, etc. Iodum and Kali iod. have caused the absorption of fluid from the tunica vaginalis and the disappearance of other symptoms of hydrocele. Mercurius is frequently indicated. Pulsatilla in lymphatic temperaments, with veins prominent, swollen and bluish in color. Rhododendron when no cause can be found. Rhus tox. when the left side is involved, while Spongia, from its pathogenesis, should be frequently indicated.

HÆMATOCELE.—This is an extravasation of blood into the tunica vaginalis, the sheath of the spermatic cord or the various structures and cellular tissue of the scrotum, producing a swelling of varying size.

Etiology.—It may be caused by rupture of a blood-vessel of the scrotum, from external violence, imperfectly ligated or overlooked vessels from surgical operation, or extravasation of blood into the tissues from blood-vessels weakened by disease.

Clinical History of Acute Hæmatocele.—It appears suddenly when resulting from traumatism or the giving way of a ligature after surgical operation, the scrotum becoming very painful from the large and rapid extravasation of blood, which may be bright red, but more often is dark brown and mixed with pus. The scrotum becomes blue-black or livid, and if the swelling is great the penis will be retracted. If the extravasation is large or suppuration has resulted, evidence of fluctuation will be present. When the hæmatocele is a complication of a cyst or hydrocele the original swelling becomes more tense and painful, accompanied by symptoms of shock, which may be followed by traumatic fever and suppuration.

The acute form of hæmatocele is differentiated from hydrocele by its history, sudden appearance, absence of translucency, and general heavy feeling of the swollen scrotum.

Treatment.—The acute hæmatocele has no tendency towards spontaneous cure, and if not relieved will increase in size. Rest and quiet are imperative with removal of the cause, cold applications, support of the scrotum, and Aconite if there is fever and shock; Arnica and Conium if the result of traumatism; and later Sulphur, Pulsatilla, Nux vomica, Hamamelis, etc. The removal of the extravasated blood from the tunica vaginalis by tapping will often be necessary, after which the cavity may be washed out with a hot, normal saline solution until the fluid comes away clear. Iodine or Carbolic acid is then injected, as directed in *hydrocele*.

When the clots are large and the tension great, or suppuration threatens, open the sac, remove the blood clots and other foreign substances and dress antiseptically.

Clinical History of Chronic Hæmatocele.—In old hæmatoceles the fibrin of the blood adheres to the walls of the tunica vaginalis or cyst, gradually thickens and becomes organized. The tumefied mass in time becomes heavy, tense and hard; this sometimes leads to the diagnosis of malignant tumor or chronic enlargement, and operation for excision has even been attempted. In these cases, in order to confirm the diagnosis, the peculiar sensitiveness of the testicle to pressure should be remembered. The testicle is usually found behind the tumor and about in the centre; sometimes it is displaced, and the sensitive point will be found elsewhere.

Always locate the position of the testicle before commencing an operation for the removal of these products of exudation, as serious injury has followed neglect of this precaution.

Hæmatocele like hydrocele is pyriform in shape, but it is not translucent and has a heavy feel. The pain varies greatly and in the most chronic may scarcely be noticed. The general health remains good. Sometimes even with the points already given it is impossible to make a diagnosis without incision or the use of the exploring trocar. When clots close the opening of the trocar or inflammation is imminent from tension, incision is the treatment indicated and should be made only under the most rigid antiseptic precautions.

When incision is indicated in hæmatocele a small opening is made with a thin bistoury high up and in front of the tumor and carried straight down the anterior surface of the scrotum by means of blunt-pointed scissors to avoid injury to the testicle. In making the incision it should always be remembered that full drainage must be provided for.

Turn out clots and wash the cavity with a hot, normal saline solution or dilute Carbolic acid and remove the damaged and redundant part. Ligate the vessels and touch the raw surfaces with a solution of Chloride of Zinc. The edges of the wound and the tunica vaginalis are then attached by sutures and the cavity packed with Iodoform gauze, which is allowed to remain until separated by exudation. Dress antiseptically until the wound is closed by granulations. Erysipelas and gangrene sometimes follow this operation in the aged from the severe and rapid reaction, hence castration is believed to be the better operation. In the young and middle-aged the operation is not only successful, but the parts are largely restored to usefulness, as the testicle is not involved in hæmatocele. Happily in the chronic cases the exhibition of Sulphur, Iodum, Kali iod., etc., often produces satisfactory results.

ENCYSTED HÆMATOCELE is an effusion of blood into an encysted hydrocele; it is of infrequent occurrence.

Treatment.—The same as that advised in *hæmatocele*.

HÆMATOCELE OF THE CORD is an effusion of blood into the cord; if general it is called diffuse hæmatocele of the cord; if into a cyst or when circumscribed it is known as encysted hæmatocele of the cord. Both conditions are rare, and only recognized by their clinical history.

Treatment.—As advised for *hæmatocele*.

INFLAMMATION OF THE TESTICLE may affect the epididymis (epididymitis) or the secreting part (orchitis) irrespective of each other as their circulation is independent; in some cases, and especially after traumatism, both may be simultaneously involved.

EPIDIDYMITIS.—Inflammation of the epididymis is characterized by rapid swelling, pain, tension and soreness of the organ.

Etiology.—Excessive venery, gleet, stricture, calcareous concretions in the prostatic portion of the urethra; acute or chronic prostatitis; gonorrhœa; the neglect to wear a properly fitting suspensory bandage or lifting during an attack of any urethral inflammation are the most frequent causes, though it may result from instrumentation and surgical operation in and around the prostate gland and neck of the bladder, traumatism and sometimes gout.

The first attack is usually the most severe; one attack predisposes to another and relapses are frequent.

Pathological Anatomy.—In all cases the tunica vaginalis is involved as it is continuous in structure with the epididymis. It is congested and inflamed, exuding serum, sero-sanguineous and plastic material into the tunica vaginalis; the tubes of the epididymis are greatly distended, with an inflammatory, plastic and homogeneous exudation. The secreting part of the testis, however, while markedly hyperæmic, rarely becomes inflamed.

Clinical History.—Epididymitis may be single or double. At first there is a slight uneasy feeling, referred to the groin, extending up to the back, as if the cord was stretched, and possibly a little fever, increased frequency of urination with pain in the perinæum and scrotum. In a few hours the parts commence to swell, with pain in proportion to the swelling, due to the effusion into and the rapid distention of the tunica vaginalis. In the more moderate cases the exudation is less, and consequently the pain is not so severe. The epididymis becomes inflamed, swollen and painful, the secreting part of the testicle lying in front of it. The pain may be of the most agonizing and sickening character, and is greatly increased by standing. The scrotum appears red, swollen and œdematous, with veins standing out tortuous and prominent. The whole organ is sore and sensitive to touch, so much so that the patient will, unconsciously to himself, support and protect it with the hand. The swelling becomes oval or irregular in shape, and may attain the size of an orange. If urethritis existed before and was the cause of the disease, the discharge will decrease or stop, to return on the cure of the epididymitis.

The disease advances rapidly for two to six days, but is generally relieved or cured in about two weeks, although an inflammatory induration of the tail of the epididymis may persist for years. This induration may, by its mere presence or future contraction, occlude, in part or entirely, the tubes of which the tail is made up; it may cause sterility if both are involved. Fortunately the occlusion is rarely complete even when the conducting tubes of both have been diseased. The testes always retain their power of secretion, even when the tubes are completely obstructed, and if, at any future period, the canal is opened the spermatozoa will again make their appearance in the seminal fluid.

Obstruction of the ducts of the epididymis does not in any way interfere with the act of copulation or ejaculation of seminal fluid, which does not contain spermatozoa. Microscopical examinations made in a large number of cases have demonstrated that in double epididymitis, when treatment is continued, the spermatozoa will again be found in the semen in from two to eight months.

The nodule in the tail of the epididymis is liable to become very sensitive and irritable, the least touch producing the most agonizing pain.

Epididymitis is sometimes accompanied by great swelling and inflammation of the spermatic cord, which may extend up into the inguinal ring; it may result in inflammatory strangulation, recognized by fever, vomiting, pain, shock, etc., and leeches or puncture of the tense and inflamed cord may be required to give relief.

Treatment.—Rest and suspension of the scrotum are the earliest requirements. If proper precautions are taken the statistical record of one case of epididymitis in every six or eight cases of gonorrhœa may be avoided. When the dragging sensation in the inguinal region and cord, pain in the perinæum and frequency of urination announce the commencement of an epididymitis it can be aborted if the testicle is properly supported, a hot bath taken, followed by rest in bed for a day or two, together with light diet and the administration of Aconite, Belladonna, Pulsatilla or Clematis, as indicated. If the inflammation continues, accompanied by increased swelling, and Belladonna, etc., does not relieve the intense pain, which often occurs in very acute cases, immediate relief can be given by puncturing the tense tunica vaginalis (under proper aseptic conditions) and allowing a little of the fluid to escape.*

* This shows that the pain in epididymitis is due to overdistention of the sac.

After the puncture, or in cases where the pain is not severe and puncture has not been necessary, the scrotum should be wrapped in cotton, covered with oiled silk and placed and retained in a shallow suspensory bandage, with side laces, to give gentle, equable and continuous pressure. This dressing gives rest, heat and pressure to the parts and allows the patient to continue at his daily vocation without loss of time. Some will not permit puncture to be made; they must remain in bed and apply hot poultices every three hours, made of tobacco and flaxseed, large enough to completely envelop the scrotum; the poultice should be covered with cotton or flannel and finally enclosed in a piece of oiled silk. To retain the poultice a bandage is tied around the body and a large silk handkerchief is folded from corner to corner, the base of the triangle placed under the scrotum and the ends tied to the bandage in the median line; the middle end or apex of the triangle is brought up and also tied to the bandage at the same point. This simple bandage supports the scrotum and enables the patient to move freely about in bed without danger of dislodging the poultice.

Hot fomentations of Hamamelis applied with absorbent cotton in the same manner as the poultice act very satisfactorily. After the pain has subsided and there is a decrease in the size of the swelling a paste, made of equal parts of extract of Belladonna and Mercurial ointment, spread upon lint, can be applied to the scrotum and retained in place by a suspensory bandage which supports the organ at the same time. Under this treatment the swelling rapidly subsides. When double epididymitis has existed it is wise to continue the Belladonna and Mercurial salve until the swelling ceases to diminish or entirely disappears, to avoid, if possible, the occlusion of the tubes in the epididymis.

Some good results have been obtained from the daily application of an ointment of Nitrate of Silver 1 to 10.

When pain has ceased, strapping is advocated by some to reduce the swelling. The hair is first removed from the scrotum, which is then made aseptic. Strips of adhesive plaster, about an inch wide and six or eight inches long, are cut. The spermatic cord is encircled about the swelling with the left hand or by an assistant to push the tumor well down into the scrotum, making the walls tense and firm. A piece of muslin bandage is now carried twice around the swollen parts at the upper border and fastened at the end by a piece of adhesive plaster. This cotton bandage prevents the adhesive straps cutting into the tissues. The straps are now applied, encircling the upper part of the scrotum, over-lapping one another from above downward, until a little below the centre, when the direction of the strap must be changed and it is carried under the scrotum so as to draw the pendulous part upward. Complete the dressing by a single strip to hold the ends.

Pain sometimes follows the strapping, but it usually passes off in an hour or so. The parts should then be supported by a suspensory bandage and the patient allowed to go about and attend to his business. Remove the straps in from twenty-four to forty-eight hours or whenever they become loose. Some œdema of the pendulous portion of the scrotum may be noticed on removal of the straps, but it is not, as a rule, of any consequence.

When the parts have been strapped and much pain follows, the straps must be removed at once, as over-tight strapping has at times caused gangrene.

Aconite will be required for the fever and arterial tension. Belladonna when the pain is excessive or neuralgic and the parts swollen and congested. Gelsemium is useful for the fever, swelling, etc., but Hamamelis and especially Pulsatilla are the remedies most frequently indicated for the active symptoms, and later, Clematis, Mercurius or Sulphur.

ORCHITIS is an inflammation of the secreting part of the testis, it may be acute or chronic.

ACUTE ORCHITIS.—Etiology.—It may be caused by malaria, but usually is the result of metastasis from parotitis in young adults.

Clinical History.—Acute orchitis may involve the epididymis. It runs a rapid course with a moderate amount of pain, swelling and fever. Recovery usually takes place in about two weeks.

Treatment.—Rest in bed, suspension of the parts with hot tobacco and flaxseed poultices, or hot fomentations.

A spray of a hot two per cent. Carbolic acid solution used for fifteen minutes daily, afterwards wrapping the parts in cotton and supporting them by a suspensory bandage is highly recommended, but it must not be continued longer than fifteen minutes, as it excoriates the skin.

Remedies.—Aconite, Belladonna, Pulsatilla, Hamamelis, Gelsemium and Quinia sulph.

CHRONIC OR TRUE ORCHITIS.—It may terminate in recovery, abscess or gangrene.

Etiology.—It may be caused by traumatism, exposure to cold, excessive venery, and in the strumous, the gouty, the debilitated and in old age, though it sometimes occurs in children.

Clinical History.—Pain referred to the lumbar region is often the only subjective symptom, but usually the pain in the testicle when it occurs is agonizing, and out of all proportion to the amount of swelling, and is due to the distention of the firm and unyielding tunica albuginea.

The pain may be continuous, gradually disappear or stop suddenly. The sudden cessation of the pain may indicate gangrene or death of the part, which will be accompanied by a chill and rapid swelling of the parts. When pus is formed it may work its way to the surface and point, when it should be opened; if it occurs in the centre of the organ it may become encapsulated.

As the disease progresses the testis becomes swollen, ovoid in form, hard, tense and sensitive, and the scrotum red, inflamed and œdematous. Examination and manipulation of the inflamed and swollen organ may be so exquisitely painful as to cause faintness, if not complete syncope.

Recovery without atrophy may occur, or the testicle may undergo degeneration, or result in the formation of an abscess with sinuses, which in time may terminate in fungous outgrowths which will necessitate the removal of the organ.

Treatment.—For the pain and acute symptoms rest in bed, suspension of the testes by a sling or suspensory bandage, with hot tobacco and flaxseed poultices. If these means do not give relief the puncture of the tunica albuginea with a sharp-pointed, narrow bistoury introduced posteriorly, under proper antiseptic conditions, usually relieves the pain and tension.

Remedies. — Conium, Pulsatilla, Gelsemium, Aurum, Clematis, Hypericum, Kali iod., Mercurius, Rhus tox., and Hepar sulph.

SYPHILITIC ORCHITIS.—Etiology.—It is developed only during an attack of constitutional syphilis.

Clinical History.—The growth is slow and painless. The testicle becomes hard, tense and nodular. It often exists a long time before it is discovered.

Treatment.—The disease is readily amenable to Mercurius and Kali iod.

HERNIA TESTIS.—This is a benign fungous growth of the testicle.

Clinical History.—These outgrowths are the natural sequence of degeneration or abscess following true orchitis. They present a granulating surface, somewhat pale in color, which bleeds slightly. Manipulation of the growth gives the peculiar sickening feeling experienced when pressure is applied to the normal testicle.

Treatment.—First make a microscopical examination to differentiate from malignant fungoid growths. Pressure and caustics often act satisfactorily. The edges can be scarified, brought together by sutures over the hernia and dressed antiseptically until union is complete.

Remedies. — Thuja, Mercurius, Calcarea carb., Baryta carb. and Nitric acid have cured this condition, but as treatment is sometimes ineffectual, castration may be required.

CYSTS OF THE TESTICLE are frequently found in or upon the testicle, either alone or associated with some other disease; they vary in size from a millet seed to an egg. At first they grow slowly, but if bruised they become inflamed and grow rapidly; sometimes suppuration occurs. They may contain watery, serous or sebaceous matter, hair, teeth, bones, etc. Pain is usually absent. If of large size they often will give fluctuation, and are sometimes mistaken for hydrocele or hæmatocele.

Treatment.—When they become large and troublesome, inflamed or suppurating, an operation will be necessary to relieve. If within the testicle, castration is indicated; if upon the side of the testicle the growths can be dissected off.

Remedies.— Apis, Conium, Graphites, Sepia, Sulphur, etc., are useful in some cases.

CANCER OF THE TESTICLE may be either of the medullary or scirrhous variety, the former being the most common. It occurs at any time of life, but more frequently in the young. The hard variety (scirrhus) is usually secondary to general carcinomatous involvement, and is usually to be traced to some traumatism. It progresses slowly, though sometimes its growth is rapid. At first the tumor is smooth and tense, from the general swelling and effusion into the tunica albuginea, but as time goes on it becomes uneven and irregular in shape. After a time spots of deep fluctuation appear, which break through the tunica albubinea giving rise to malignant fungoid growths, with a bloody, ichorous discharge. The veins of the scrotum become prominent and swollen and the legs œdematous. The abdominal, pelvic and inguinal glands become enlarged and infiltrated with cancerous material. The growth increases rapidly, accompanied by sharp shooting and burning pains. When a question of diagnosis exists, always confirm with the microscope. The duration of the disease is about two years.

Treatment.—In the early history Arsenicum or Conium may prove useful, but castration is usually necessary.

TUBERCULAR TESTIS.—There are two varieties, the true and the false.

THE FALSE OR PSEUDO-TUBERCULAR TESTIS is recognized as a slow inflammatory condition involving the epididymis and sometimes extending to the neighboring parts.

Etiology.—Chronic urethral discharges are the principal cause.

Clinical History.—Small nodular swellings appear in and on the epididymis, which grow very slowly without pain or special discomfort. The vas deferens may become involved. These nodules are liable to break down into abscesses, and by adhesive inflammation with the scrotal tissues allow the pus to discharge externally, leaving an indolent sinus which may result in a fungous growth. The lymphatic glands are not involved as in cancer.

Treatment.—That given for the true variety together with the internal administration of Spongia, Aurum, Calcarea carb., Mercurius bin-iodide, Silicea, Hepar sulph. and Sulphur.

TRUE TUBERCULAR TESTIS.—This is a most serious disease, coming on insidiously without apparent cause unless associated with general tuberculosis. This disease is most common in the young.

Pathological Anatomy.—Examination reveals the fact that the tubercles are developed in the lymph canals and in the connective tissue around the seminal tubes and ducts. They coalesce and form dirty yellow masses which break down into a cheesy material, and finally develop into abscesses; they are not encapsulated but are in direct relation to the surrounding tissue.

Clinical History.—It may be preceded by a slight urethral discharge which has had no apparent cause and which may stop of itself. It is occasionally accompanied by a little vesical irritability. The disease is not painful, and therefore may go on for some time without being discovered; in fact, the testicle early in the disease loses its sensibility, and when examined does not give the usual sickening sensation even if handled roughly. The growth never attains any great size; it always commences in the epididymis then involves the vas deferens, seminal vesicles and finally the testis proper, thus differing from chronic orchitis, which begins in the testis and rarely involves the epididymis.

On examination the epididymis will be found hard, knotty, irregular and swollen, with heaviness and fullness. There will be no lymphatic enlargement or increase in the size of the veins, as occurs in cancer. One or both testicles may be involved, hence the sexual appetite will be lost or impaired in proportion to the pathological change in the testes. As the disease progresses one or more of the nodules may become painful, swollen and inflamed; an abscess forms, which often burrows outward through the tissues that have been the seat of adhesive inflammation and discharges a thick creamy material and sinus will remain through which other nodules will discharge. It may granulate or form a hernia testis.

Treatment.—If suppuration has begun and abscess is inevitable, poultice, open and curette. Nourishing diet and change of air.

Remedies.—Aurum, Spongia, Mercurius, etc.; if these are not successful castration is often advisable.

CASTRATION.—Professor Helmuth's suggestions in this operation are undoubtedly important. After the patient is anæsthetized and all proper aseptic and antiseptic precautions observed, the cord is taken between the thumb and index finger of the left hand, just at its exit from the external abdominal ring, and the integument having been rendered tense by firm pressure, an acupressure pin is introduced at right angles to the cord, the head of the pin is depressed and the point brought out on the opposite side. To make the operation still more safe he introduces another pin about half an inch below and places over them, in order to hold the cord in position and prevent retraction, two small india rubber rings. An incision is made on the anterior aspect of the scrotum, extending from the external abdominal ring to the bottom of the scrotum, then dissect out the glands and divide the cord with a single stroke of the knife. There will be no retraction of the cord and no bleeding. The cremasteric, spermatic and artery of the vas deferens must be tied separately and bleeding points secured. Then dress antiseptically and leave proper drainage.

NEURALGIA OF THE TESTIS.—Sometimes designated as irritable testicle. It may attack one or both.

Etiology.—It occurs with or without appreciable lesion of the testis or cord, from atrophy or hypertophy of the testes, hydrocele, varicocele, reflex from deep urethral, prostatic and bladder diseases. It may be associated with nodular growths on the epididymis, and may accompany a nephritic colic. It is sometimes caused by the spasmodic contraction of the cremaster muscles, associated with vomiting, cold sweat, etc., and from continence in widowers, and from sudden reformation in the masturbator; malaria, gout and syphilis often produce neuralgia of the testes.

Clinical History.—The pain varies in intensity, sometimes being greatly increased by the slightest touch; it may be continuous, spasmodic, localized or radiating over various parts of the body, and often become so severe as to cause collapse.

Treatment.—Massage, general hygiene, cold applications, etc.

Remedies.—If from perverted sexual functions, Ignatia. Neuralgic pain, heat and over-sensitiveness of the parts, Hamamelis. When accompanied by hard and indurated growths, Aurum. Neuralgic pains with or without cause, Magnesium phos. or Colocynthis.

VARICOCELE is recognized by the elongation and enlargement of the veins of the spermatic cord. It is the most common affection of the male genito-urinary organs and may be found to a greater or less degree in ten per cent. of the male population.

Etiology.—It may be caused by anything which increases the flow of blood through the veins of the testicle or cord and interferes with the return circulation, as over-exercise, standing, long marches, constipation, constriction of the parts by the clothing, and over-lifting. It frequently occurs as the result of perverted sexual functions or habits, either over-indulgence or unsatisfied longing, which causes passive and continuous congestion of the parts.

Clinical History.—It occurs almost exclusively on the left side, due to the anatomical construction of the parts. It is not necessarily associated with venous enlargement elsewhere; in fact, they bear no relation to one another. It is essentially a disease of early life, being found in infancy, and commencing almost invariably before the twenty-fifth year. It may exist for years unnoticed; its progress is slow and irregular. Frequently, after reaching a certain point, the condition remains stationary without treatment and often without cause; again, as after an epididymitis, it may increase rapidly. In this disease there is pain, discomfort and dragging, referred to the scrotum, perinæum, cord and back, but the pain is never in proportion to the size of the varicocele. It is sometimes associated with neuralgia of the testicle. The dilatation of the veins varies from a slight turgescence and enlargement to enormous distention, elongation and thickening of their coats, with destruction of the valves. The varicocele, when of large size, appear as a pyriform tumor encroaching on the opposite side of the scrotum, and the bluish color of the venous blood in the enlarged veins may sometimes be seen through the scrotal tissues.

When manipulated, the veins within the scrotum feel like bunches of angle-worms or cords. If any doubt exists as to the diagnosis, the patient should be placed in a recumbent position and the scrotum elevated, when the tumor can be easily reduced; then make pressure at the inguinal ring and request the patient to stand. If the pressure is strong enough to compress the artery there will be no change, but if the pressure is lessened, so as to compress the veins only, the scrotum will gradually fill up and become distended from below upwards as the blood is brought in by the artery. The superficial veins of the scrotal walls are also enlarged. When the varicocele is marked there is usually some atrophy of the testicle.

Treatment.—Traumatic cases and those of moderate severity are best treated by frequent cold sponging of the scrotum and supporting the parts with a suspensory bandage. Marriage is to be recommended when the trouble arises from perverted sexual functions.

The more severe cases, while not endangering life, may require operation. Dr. Keyes' is the best. The scrotum is first washed with a Bichloride of Mercury solution 1 to 1000. The patient stands beside the bed, so that if he becomes faint, which often happens after the puncture, he may at once be placed upon his back and the operation continued in that position. The distended veins are separated by manipulation from the vas deferens, and can be easily felt among the different structures of the cord, and are moved towards the outer side of the scrotum. The Keyes' varicocele needle, (fig. 37)

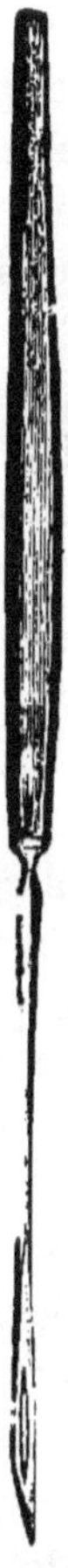

FIG. 37.

is threaded with one strand of silk and made to transfix the scrotum between the veins and the vas deferens. When the eye of the needle emerges on the opposite side of the scrotum the silk is drawn through the eye with a teriaculum and disengaged. The punctured scrotum is then traversed independently by the needle and one strand of silk. The scrotum is again washed with the bichloride solution and the needle partly withdrawn until it clears the veins without allowing it to emerge at the original point of entrance. The veins are now allowed to rejoin the vas deferens, and the point of the needle is again advanced upon the outer side of the veins under the dartos and made to emerge posteriorly at the exact point where the silk is protruding. The eye of the needle is then opened, the silk placed in it and the instrument entirely withdrawn, carrying the silk with it.

The scrotum is again washed, the hair is removed from the posterior point of puncture on the scrotum, and the anterior ends of the silk being firmly held, the scrotum is pulled away so that the shreds of dartos included in the loop at the posterior puncture may be pulled free from the integument. Remove all hairs at the anterior point of puncture to avoid their being tied in; forcibly tie the silk with a triple knot for security. Cut the ends short and let the knot sink into the scrotum. Bleeding seldom occurs. Oozing at the punctured spot is simply dusted with Iodoform or Iodol.

Dress with absorbent cotton and support the parts in a sling. Pain and swelling sometimes follow this operation but as soon as the patient is able to stand he is allowed to go about, usually after the third day. The hard spot remains at the point of ligature for a year, and possibly longer.

Remedies—Arnica, when traumatism has been the cause of the varicocele. Aconite, if accompanied by fever and engorgement of the vessels. Hamamelis is one of the most important remedies in this condition; it has cured many cases of varicocele; testicles swollen, with drawing pain in the spermatic cord; organs greatly relaxed and perspiring, with darting pains from the scrotum to the abdomen. Lachesis when the veins assume a livid appearance, accompanied by mental depression. Nux vomica, when associated with gout, constipation, gastric derangements and irritability and when excesses have been the cause. Pulsatilla, the veins appear blue with painful drawing, lasting a long time, in the spermatic cord, which is swollen, painful, etc. Sulphur is frequently beneficial; the testicles hang down relaxed with soreness and moisture of the scrotum.

CHAPTER XV.
SPECIAL THERAPY FOR SCROTAL DISEASES.

Acid. Nitricum.—Orchitis. Hernia testis. Hard nodules on scrotum suppurating. Sore, itching spots on scrotum. Swelling of scrotum sensitive to touch. Bruised, transitory, burning pain in testicles. Tearing pain in spermatic cord.

Acid. Oxalicum.—Terrible neuralgic pain in spermatic cord; worse from slightest motion.

Aconite.—Acute orchitis. Epididymitis and varicocele. Acute inflammation of the testes, caused by cold or gonorrhœa, with tearing and bruised feeling. Testes swollen, hard, with drawing pains. Engorgement of the vessels. High fever, full pulse, restlessness, anxiety, agonizing pain.

Agnus Castus.—Chronic orchitis. Atrophy. Great relaxation and coldness of the testes and scrotum. Crawling sensation in the testes. Loss of sexual power.

Apis.— Cystic growths. Hydrocele. Epididymitis. Erysipelatous inflammation of the scrotum. Excessive œdema of the scrotum. Testes swollen, with tension and itching. Fullness, with aching and stinging pains. Scrotum tense, full, swollen and œdematous.

Argentum Nitricum.—Neuralgia. Epididymitis. Orchitis. Spasmodic contraction of the cremaster muscle, drawing up the testis. Right testicle enlarged, hard. Bruised pains. Pain as from pins and needles in right testicle. Pain shooting down cord and into testicle. Orchitis from suppressed gonorrhœa. Genitals shrivelled, with loss of desire.

Arnica.—Contusions and bruises of the genital organs. Testicle swollen, indurated and tender.

Arsenicum.—Hernia testis. Scrotum swollen. Hydrocele of children. Testes swollen. Cutting colic. Cramplike pain at abdominal ring and perinæum. Hydrocele in weak and debilitated patients. Fungoid growths, burning pains, with acrid, burning, corrosive discharge.

Aurum Met.—Orchitis, chronic or tubercular. Neuralgia. Induration of the testicle, with pressive pain on touch. Testes swollen, indurated, with severe tensive pain, especially at night. Aching as if bruised. Hydrocele. Testes on the point of atrophy. False tuberculosis of testes. Low-spirited, lifeless, loss of memory, etc. Neuralgic pain in the cord with swollen testicle.

Baryta Carb.—Hernia testis. Senile orchitis.

Belladonna.— Epididymitis. Orchitis. Neuralgia. Acute inflammation of the testes with much swelling and induration. Pain unbearable, neuralgic in character. Great sensitiveness. Scrotum hot and swollen. Tendency to congestion of the brain and delirium. Stitching and throbbing pains. Tearing in left spermatic cord from below upwards in the evening or when falling asleep, with sharp lancinating pain in the testicles.

Bromium.—Testicles swollen hard and perfectly smooth. Pain increased from jarring. Parts hot and inflamed. To be considered in persons of light complexion and blue eyes.

Calcarea Carb. — Adapted to scrofulous patients.

Scrotum relaxed. Crushing, pressive and bruised pain in testes. Pain in spermatic cord as if contracted.

Carbo Veg.—Swelling and hardness of the testes. Hernia testis.

Clematis.—Epididymitis. Orchitis. Neuralgia. Painful swelling and inflammation of both testes. Pains shoot from testicles up the spermatic cord. Testicles swollen, indurated, heavy and hang down. Pinching and bruised pain in testicle on touch, with drawing and tensive pains in the inguinal region, thigh and scrotum. Pain drawing and shooting upward in the spermatic cord. Pain is worse at night and from warmth. Inflammation sub-acute in character. Epididymitis from gonorrhœa.

Colocynthis.—Painful twinges and drawing pain in testicle. Neuralgia of the testicle.

Cannabis Sativa.—Dragging sensation; pulling and pressure on standing. Epididymis and spermatic cord swollen in spots, like soft beans. Tensive pains in spermatic cord.

Capsicum.—Scrotum seems cold. Tendency to atrophy of the testes. Drawing pains in the spermatic cord, with pain in the testicles during and after urinating.

China.—Spermatic cord, testes and epididymis painful and swollen. Tearing pains worse on the left side, especially in the evening. Chronic orchitis, with general weakness and debility.

Conium.—Orchitis from injury. Induration and swelling of the testes. Scrotum swollen. Cutting, griping, sticking pains in the testes. Drawing pain in spermatic cord. Testes heavy and sore. Pain in testicles after erection.

Gelsemium.—Epididymitis from gonorrhœa or exposure to wet or cold.

Graphites.—Swollen testes. Hydrocele, accompanied by general scrofulous disease, skin eruptions and constipation.

Hamamelis.—Varicocele. Epididymitis. Neuralgia. Soreness, great pain and swelling of testes. Spermatic veins enlarged, swollen and inflamed. Drawing pains in spermatic cord. Neuralgic pains from testicles up the cord to the stomach, worse at night and in rainy weather. Pain in spermatic cord, running into testicles. Dull, heavy pains in testicles. Pain almost unbearable at times in the scrotum, which is red, hot and shining. Perspiration and moisture on scrotum.

Hepar Sulph.—Abscess and hernia testis, with usual symptoms of commencing suppuration.

Iodum.—Orchitis. Testes diminished in size and consistency, with loss of sexual power. Burning pain in right side of scrotum. Dragging pain toward testicle. Testes hypertrophied, with pain, extending towards abdomen. Hydrocele has been cured by this remedy.

Kali Carb.—Soreness of the scrotum with bruised feeling. Swelling of testicles and spermatic cord. Tension in left testicle. Spasmodic contraction of spermatic cords.

Kali Iod.—Chronic specific orchitis.

Lycopodium.—Orchitis. Scrotum relaxed even during copulation. Jerking, stinging, sticking, griping and pinching pains in testicles. Drawing and sticking pains in seminal ducts. Impotence.

Mercurius.—Sub-acute epididymitis. Orchitis, simple, tubercular or specific. Testicles swollen hard. Scrotum shining, with dragging, drawing and itching pains. Drawing pain in groins. Spasmodic tearing between testicles. Sensation of coldness of the testicles. When abscess threatens and there is chilliness and perspiration. Pains are worse at night.

Mercurius Bin-iod.—Syphilitic orchitis. Testicle and spermatic cord sensitive.

Nux Vomica.—Stitching, aching and contractive pain in the testicle. Pinching and itching in the scrotum. Tearing in the spermatic cord. Gouty diathesis.

Phytolacca.—Epididymitis. Acute and chronic orchitis. Sharp, griping pains shooting up the spermatic cord. Paroxysmal pains followed by soreness.

Pulsatilla.—Epididymitis. Orchitis. Varicocele. Dark-red, painful swelling of testicles and spermatic cord, especially if caused by gonorrhœa or metastasis from parotitis. Pressive, tensive, tearing pains. Testicles so sore that the touch of the clothing cannot be tolerated. Drawing pains, lasting a long time, in the spermatic cord. The veins bluish, with soreness and tingling pain. Pain may shoot to the back or down the thighs. No thirst with fever. Especially adapted to those of lymphatic temperament.

Rhododendron.—Epididymitis. Hydrocele. Testicle indurated, distressing pains in epididymis. Testes drawn up, swollen and painful. Swelling and induration with drawing pains shooting to thigh and abdomen. Testicle tends to atrophy. Feeling as if the testicle had been crushed. Constrictive drawing pains in the testicles (alternately). Sticking and drawing pain in the right testicle and spermatic cord, especially at night.

Sepia.—Drawing, cutting, pinching rheumatic pains in the testicle. Heat in the scrotum. Pains extend into the thighs.

Silicea.—Elephantiasis of scrotum. Hydrocele. Scrotum itching and moist. Pain in testicle at night and when lying down. Testicle indurated, with compressive, distending, jerking pain. Crawling pain in testicle. Pressure in spermatic cords. Abscess and hernia testis.

Spongia.—Orchitis. Acute, chronic or tubercular hydrocele. Testicle smooth, swollen and inflamed. Squeezing, strangulating and aching pains in testicle. Testes swollen hard, with throbbing, dull stitches and darting pains shooting up the spermatic cord. Testis painful to touch, squeezing pain in testes and cord, worse on motion of the body or contact with clothes.

Staphisagria.—Drawing, tearing pain in right testicle. Swollen testes from metastatic parotitis. Drawing, burning, stitching pain from right inguinal region in spermatic cord to testicle. Aching in left testicle when walking; worse from touch.

Sulphur.—Testicles relaxed and hang down. Moisture on the scrotum. Pressure and tension in the spermatic cord. Induration of the testicle. Tingling in testicle.

Thuja.—Enlargement of veins of epididymis. Aching pains in testicles as if crushed, aggravated by motion. Sharp stitches extending into spermatic cord. Hernia testis. Sticking and boring pain in scrotum and spermatic cord. Itching, crawling and burning pain in scrotum.

Veratrum Viride.—Neuralgia of the testes. Acute orchitis. Erysipelatous swelling of scrotum. Testicle swollen, pain shooting from testicle up the spermatic cord. High fever and arterial tension.

CHAPTER XVI.

FUNCTIONAL DISEASES OF THE GENITAL ORGANS.

IMPOTENCE is the inability to accomplish the sexual act, due to some abnormal condition of the economy, although when the erection is sufficient to make an intromission with a discharge of fluid they are potent.

Impotence when due to a pathological condition is of the true variety; if it arises from nervous conditions or functional disturbances without pathological change it is false impotence.

TRUE IMPOTENCE may be partial or complete. The complete may be congenital or acquired, as when it arises from lack of development, hypertrophy, hydrocele, varicocele, scrotal hernia, etc., or from change in form following injury, surgical operations and reflex from cerebral or spinal injury or disease.

Complete impotence is rare. The partial form is frequent and is usually associated with some pathological condition of the prostatic urethra. Hyperæmia or inflammatory conditions here seem to produce a profound action upon the spinal motor centres. If the reflex excitement of the genito-spinal centre is abolished it produces an atonic condition which not only interferes with the vigor but also the duration of the sexual act, even without local urethral lesions.

The causes of the pathological change in the prostatic urethra are many, the most important undoubtedly being the extension of a gonorrhœal urethritis which has been neglected, prolonged sexual excitement without gratification, perverted sexual acts and excesses; varicocele, irritation of the glans penis, strictures, etc. In all cases we should endveavor to find the cause and remove it when possible.

Treatment.—The examination of the patient must be methodical and complete. Deformities must be corrected by the proper surgical treatment. The urethra must be explored by means of the bulbous bougie or the Otis urethrometer. When a stricture is found it must be relieved by the indicated surgical treatment, as this condition is a special cause of continued urethral congestion. When there is a contracted meatus, phimosis or varicocele, operation often proves very beneficial. If due to perverted sexual habits these must be corrected, lewd thoughts must not be indulged in, and anything which tends to excite the sexual appetite should be avoided. Books of travel and of general interest must be their sole reading, with proper hygiene and out-door employment. If there is evidence of a pathological condition in the prostatic urethra it should be toned up by the introduction every third day of a full-sized cold steel sound, which can pass the normal meatus without pain or annoyance, or a hollow sound which allows hot or cold water to flow through it, making local application of heat or cold, as best suited to the case, may be used for ten minutes every third day. The water may be either at a temperature of 40° or 106° F.

If erosions or marked hyperæsthesia of the prostatic urethra are present, inject with a deep urethral syringe from 2 to 8 drops of a solution of Nitrate of Silver, 8 to 20 grains to the ounce of distilled water, or 10 to 20 minims of a solution of Nitrate of Silver 1 to 2000.

Faradism often gives good results, one electrode being introduced into the prostatic urethra and the other applied to the back or perinæum, or one electrode is applied to the back or perinæum and the other to the external pendulous portion of the penis.

Daily rectal enemas of two or more quarts of hot water, thrown forcibly against the rectal wall opposite the prostate, with free exit for the water to avoid distending the rectum, have given good results. Spraying the perinæum daily, alternately with hot and cold water, has been recommended.

Remedies.—If due to a fall or blow, Arnica or Hypericum; if from syphilis, Mercurius or Kali-iod.; from sexual excesses, Phosphorus or Phosphoric acid. Unknown causes may require Agnus castus, Selenium, Arsenicum, Chininum sulph., Nux vomica, Ignatia, etc. Cures have been reported following the hypodermic injections of Spermine.

In all cases endeavor to turn the patient's mind away from himself and encourage him freely. Interdict or regulate sexual intercourse for at least six months. It is rare that these means fail to bring the patient up to a normal condition, although the sexual power varies greatly in different individuals. What would be normal in one would be excess in another. It should be remembered that there is a tendency to a decline in sexual power and desire after the fortieth year, and at the age of sixty to seventy it is frequently lost, though some have retained their sexual power and vigor until past ninety.

If the treatment proves unsuccessful, the overdistention of the prostatic urethra with Thompson's divulsor will sometimes produce the desired result.

FALSE OR NERVOUS IMPOTENCE occurs without pathological lesion.

Etiology.—It is purely of nervous origin, and may be caused by fright, anger, shame, joy, over-excitement, grief, disgust, repugnance or want of affection. Engrossing thoughts sometimes prevent perfect sexual intercourse, or it may be due to some morbid, unsatisfied fancy, the patient finding himself unable to accomplish the act except when the woman is dressed in a certain manner or is of a certain complexion, etc.

Clinical History.—The cases which cause the most annoyance and anxiety are those of young men, generally correct in their habits or who possibly have masturbated a little, when approaching a woman of questionable character suddenly find themselves unable, from over-excitement, to accomplish the sexual act. Probably they have had an occasional nocturnal pollution, and when in the company of women a slight prostatic oozing may have occurred. Their mind becomes possessed with the idea that they are impotent; they consequently become victims of melancholia from long brooding over their imaginary troubles.

Treatment.—The utmost care and attention should be given early to this class of cases. Gain their confidence, and with the proper treatment the most satisfactory results will be obtained.

Examine the parts carefully, as directed in true impotence, and if anything abnormal is found treat the condition as indicated. Out-door employment and exercise, attendance at the theatre, general increase of the bodily strength by athletic games and sponge baths, should be advised.

Insist on sexual hygiene and encourage continence. If marriage is contemplated encourage the idea, telling the patient that he will be cured before the event. At all times remember that you must treat a diseased mind.

Remedies.—Anacardium, Ignatia, Nux vom., Staphisagria, etc.

STERILITY is the inability to procreate one's kind; it may accompany impotence. It is due to the absence or a diseased condition of the spermatozoa.

Aspermatism is a condition where copulation is not completed by the ejaculation of seminal fluid. In these cases the sexual desire may be normal or absent. In some a nervous form of this condition exists where the patient is unable to complete the act except with certain parties. This condition may be due to the turning back of the seminal fluid into the bladder by spasmodic or organic stricture of the membranous urethra, stricture of any part of the urethra, stricture or fistulæ of the seminal ducts, to loss of tone of the muscles concerned in the act of ejaculation or from anæsthesia of the prostatic urethra or glans penis. In some cases it occurs without local pathological cause, due to want of lumbar reflex in the ejaculatory centres.

Azoöspermism is a condition where the seminal fluid does not contain spermatozoa, or if present they are diseased and unproductive. This may be due to double occluding epididymitis, simple, syphilitic or tubercular orchitis, obstruction at any point of the conducting tubes of both sides, atrophy or absence of the testes, etc.

Sterility may be due to want of life and tone in the spermatozoa ejected; is often the result of neurasthenia, masturbation or unnatural and ungratified sexual desire. Healthy spermatozoa should retain their life and vibratory motion for at least twelve hours after emission.

Treatment.—If due to stricture or anæsthesia of the

deep urethra, the passage of a full-sized steel sound every fourth day is indicated. The direct application of from 2 to 8 drops of a solution of Nitrate of Silver, ½ to 60 grains to the ounce, to the prostatic urethra by means of the deep urethral syringe is often followed by good results. In the syphilitic form, anti-syphilitic remedies are necessary. When from epididymitis of both sides the treatment for that disease may give satisfactory results. If from malignant or tubercular disease the treatment is unsatisfactory. When the trouble arises from stricture, and the seminal fluid is discharged after relaxation of the parts, surgical treatment may be required. Faradism should be employed when the condition is of nervous origin as recommended under impotence.

Remedies. — Damiana, Strychnia, Quinia, Iodum, Conium, etc.

Misemission is the condition where seminal fluid is ejaculated during the act without being deposited in the female organs so as to come in contact with the ovum. It may be due to hypospadias or epispadias or strictures and fistulæ of the urethra. The treatment is surgical.

MASTURBATION.—This is the production of a carnal orgasm by unnatural means. The vice is not confined to mankind, but it is practiced by the lower animals, as the monkey, horse, etc. Both male and female indulge in this pernicious habit, the former most frequently, as they possess an instinctive passion, which in the female is, as a rule, acquired only by education.

The causes are numerous, the most frequent being the intimate association with older children, who teach the habit to the younger. It may originate spontaneously from some abnormal irritation of the parts, as a long prepuce, acid or diabetic urine, etc. In the female it may arise from menstrual or leucorrhœal discharges, which have led to the handling of the genitals, and a pleasurable sensation having been produced is kept up without their knowing the harm which is being done. Other cases have resulted from the handling of children by nurses when putting them to sleep. It is said that most men have at some time or other masturbated to some extent. The practice is common at puberty, but in some way or other it becomes known that it is considered injurious to body and mind and the practice is abandoned. There is no doubt that in some cases it has produced serious results due to the excessive, unsatisfied and incomplete act, especially is this so on account of its frequent repetition. It not only acts to the detriment of the body, but it results in a depraved state of the mind if long continued. Those who discontinue the habit when they become acquainted with its iniquity escape without apparent bad results.

Those who have carried the habit to excess and continued it may be found among the circumcised as well as the uncircumcised.

Clinical History.—Careful observation will detect a tendency to pull or handle the parts. This is associated with languor and heaviness; the society of the opposite sex is avoided, as a rule, but this is more marked in the male.

The patients will be found moping around the house; they have a sheepish expression, with deep-seated eyes and lack of frankness and brightness of expression. The palms of the hands are cold and damp, the circulation poor, and the skin pale. Ambition and courage are absent and a mean-spirited condition is apparent. Impaired memory, imbecility, epilepsy, etc., may be the outcome of the vice.

Treatment.—All close friendships should be severed. The society of the opposite sex should be cultivated as much as possible. The patients' condition should be explained to them as well as the moral and physical injury which will result from the continuance of the pernicious habit. See that their sleeping room is cool, well aired and provided with a hard bed and light covering. Cold sponge baths with plenty of out-door exercise are beneficial. When the means of the patient permits advise travel. Remove all source of irritation and elevate as much as possible the moral tone. Those too young to reason with should be watched with special care; it may even become necessary to tie their hands when in bed.

Remedies.—Staphisagria, Picric acid, Calcarea carb., Nux vomica, China, Calcarea phos., Phosphoric acid, Kali brom, etc.

SATYRIASIS.—It is a morbid and excessive desire for, and an indulgence in sexual intercourse, with or without erection, leading sometimes to positive indecency. Fortunately this condition is rare; it is sometimes a symptom of brain disease.

Treatment.—If from local irritation, Cantharis; from alcoholic excesses, Nux vomica; when from brain or nervous disorders, Phosphorus and Picric acid.

NYMPHOMANIA.—This is to the female what Satyriasis is to the male. It may be caused by pruritus vulvæ, endometritis, ovaritis etc. It may be the result of ill-directed education and thought or from structural brain disorders. In the majority of these cases examination will reveal hypertrophy of the nymphæ, vaginismus and chronic follicular vulvitis. They are usually idle and over-fed. Their condition and acts may cause much annoyance and distress both to themselves and their friends.

Treatment.—Local conditions must receive proper care and the removal of the clitoris and ovaries may sometimes be required. Moral and religious influences must be brought to bear on the patient and her mind turned to healthier channels of thought and healthy occupation. Sensualities and sedentary habits must be avoided and healthy occupation and recreation insisted upon.

Remedies.—Platina, Gratiola, Origanum, Hyoscyamus, Stramonium and Tarantula Hisp.

PRIAPISM may depend upon an unbalanced nervous

condition. Reflex conditions from astigmatism, an elongated prepuce, accumulation of smegma behind the glans penis, phimosis, and stone in the bladder are frequent causes during childhood. It sometimes occurs in the later stages of eruptive diseases, in hydrophobia and tetanus, injury to or tumors of the spinal cord, cerebellum, or pons varolii, over-loading of the lower bowel, hæmorrhoids, diseases of the rectum and bladder, and especially diseases of the prostate in those advanced in years; Cantharides and other drugs in toxic doses have produced this condition.

Clinical History.—Erections of the penis become continuous or excessively prolonged. Sexual desire may be normal, increased or diminished, with or without emission, and possibly associated with an erotic mental condition. If long continued it may produce much suffering.

Treatment depends greatly upon the cause. When due to pathological lesions remove them, if possible, by the proper treatment, which is greatly aided and, if purely symptomatic, cured by Picric acid, Nux vomica, Platina, Cantharis, Phosphorus, Kali brom., Lupulin, Hyoscyamus, Belladonna or Camphor.

POLLUTIONS AND SPERMATORRHŒA.

A **Pollution** consists of an ejaculatory discharge of seminal fluid with some orgasm, occurring at night or during the day.

Spermatorrhœa is the involuntary discharge of spermatozoa, without orgasm.

POLLUTIONS become disease only when excessive. The line of demarcation between a healthy over-flow and a diseased condition is sometimes very difficult to draw, but if pollutions do not occur oftener than twice a week and the general health remains good, they may be disregarded.

The number and frequency of the nocturnal emissions varies according to the mental chastity and sexual individuality. They may occur frequently in widowerhood and in the unmarried, from continence. The emissions usually occur towards morning, when they awaken to find themselves lying on the back, with distended bladder, etc. When excessive, occurring one or more times nightly, followed by weakness, lassitude and headache, from vesical irritation or congestion of the prostatic urethra, brought on by masturbation, excessive venery, etc., this condition constitutes disease, and requires treatment.

Diurnal pollutions are of rare occurrence. They are caused by over-sensitiveness or irritability of the prostatic urethra, due to excessive venery or masturbation. The sight of some women, or some part of a woman's attire and irritation of the parts produced by the clothing, sometimes cause complete or partial emissions.

Treatment.—When nocturnal pollutions are frequent, local, general and remedial treatment are required. If there is prostatic irritability, a full-sized steel sound should be introduced from every third day to once a week, or from 3 to 5 drops of a solution of Nitrate of Silver, twenty to thirty grains to the ounce of water, may be instilled into the prostatic urethra every four to seven days. The muscular system must be developed, and exercise should be carried somewhat to excess so as to increase the tendency to sound and natural sleep. Cold baths and douches followed by dry friction of the skin are very beneficial. Heavy meals should not be partaken of late in the day. The bladder must be emptied whenever awakening during the night. A towel tied around the waist and knotted at the back will cause awakening when the dorsal position is assumed. With these means, and chaste thoughts, the appropriate remedies, Phosphoric acid, Cantharis, Kali brom., Digitalin, China, Phosphorus, Picric acid and Cimicifuga (10 to 30 drops of the tincture after meals) will usually effect a cure.

SPERMATORRHŒA.—Etiology.—The most frequent cause is undoubtedly excessive and long continued masturbation, and anything producing congestion and inflammation of the prostatic urethra as balanatis, a long prepuce, phimosis, urethritis, rectal diseases, varicocele, constipation, excessive venery, and especially where dyspeptic disorders or excessive nervous conditions exist which greatly contribute to the origin and continuance of the disease. This disorder must not, however, be confounded with a simple discharge from the urethra, in which spermatozoa are absent and which is a symptom of prostatitis, stricture, gleet, etc. These cases of false spermatorrhœa are of frequent occurrence, and it will be with the greatest difficulty that the patient can be convinced that he is not suffering from true spermatorrhœa, even when the microscope fails to find spermatozoa in the discharge.

Clinical History.—Spermatorrhœa is characterized by the involuntary discharge of seminal fluid from the urethra without carnal excitement. The discharge of seminal fluid may occur while straining at stool, from riding in a carriage or when urinating, the spermatic fluid and spermatozoa having been turned back into the bladder between the acts of micturition, passing with the urine.

Sexual vigor may be normal or excessive, but usually there is a loss of sexual vitality, the testes becoming shrunken, cold, tender and neuralgic, accompanied with coldness and retraction of the penis.

Spermatorrhœa may occur at any period of life and is usually associated with dyspeptic symptoms, pain in the back and perinæum, frequently extending into the thighs, listlessness, indifference, apathy, dull, confused feeling in the head, melancholia, neuralgia, anæmia, etc. The sufferer loses his nerve power and becomes truly an object of pity, and while he insists that he cannot be cured and has lost all hope he is forever grasping at straws. Emaciation, and hypochondriasis soon follow, nocturnal pollutions become more frequent and true impotence and sterility result.

The seminal discharge is thin, blue and the spermatozoa may be absent, or if present they show no signs of life.

Treatment.—Improvement and sometimes cure can be promised. The general and local treatment advised under pollutions are all applicable to this condition. When the parts are irritable and emissions are frequent, sitz baths at 90° to 98° F. or 50° to 70° F., as adapted to the individual case, and continued from 5 to 20 minutes at bed time, will be beneficial. Cures have been reported as the result of hypodermic injections of Spermine.

Remedies.—Conium, Digitalin, Kali brom., Phosphoric acid, Nux vomica, Canth., Ferrum brom. and China.

CHAPTER XVII.

SPECIAL THERAPY FOR FUNCTIONAL DISORDERS OF THE GENERATIVE ORGANS.

Acid Phosphoric.—Spermatorrhœa. Pollutions. Impotence. Appetite impaired. Emissions frequent from excessive venery. Emissions day or night at stool or when urinating. Whole system greatly prostrated, genital organs relaxed, flabby and hang down. Erections are absent or imperfect, ejaculation too early in the act. Feels dizzy, as if he would fall, or when reclining as though his feet would go higher than his head. Burning in the spine. Sensitive spots on the spinal column. No marked local pain. Legs weak, he totters when he walks.

Acid Picric.—Satyriasis. Pollutions. Priapism, penis erected and distended to bursting. Agonizing erection and great desire for an embrace. Seminal emission followed by exhaustion, occipital headache. Rapid development of boils over the body. Aching in the lumbar region. Numbness, crawling, and pricking in the limbs. Brain fag.

Agnus Castus.—Impotence. Sexual organs relaxed

and cold, nothing excites an erection. Sexual desire greatly diminished. Aversion to coition. Involuntary emission during the night, even after coition; discharge from the urethra watery or yellow. Emission of mucus from the urethra during sexual excitement.

Ambergris.—Awakening with violent erections without desire, the parts being externally numb after relaxation of the erection. Tingling in fore part of urethra.

Anacardium.—Loss of confidence. Discharge of prostatic or seminal fluid at stool or during micturition.

Arnica.—Impotence when there is a history of a blow or fall.

Arsenicum.—True impotence. Loss of power with strong desire. Emission with voluptuous dreams. Exhausted constitutions.

Baryta carb.—Diminished sexual power and desire. Loss of memory. Vertigo; loss of self-confidence. Feeling miserable; great debility; sensitiveness to cold. Trembling when standing and fear of falling.

Bovista.—Sexual desire increased. Frequently emission after coition. Vertigo and confusion of the mind.

Caladium.—Lewd thoughts without erections. Emissions after micturition or in dreams. Relaxation of penis during excitement and desire. Erection suddenly ceased during coition, did not know whether there was an emission. No orgasm, penis less hard than usual.

Calcarea Carb.—Impotence. Sexual power diminished, emission too quick. Great prostration after coition followed by trembling and weakness. Nervous relaxation, faintness, depression, ill-humor, weakness of memory, confusion of ideas, anxiety, face pale with dark circles around the eyes, palpitation of the heart.

Calcarea Phos.—Emissions with great weakness. Nymphomania with heat and weight in the vertex, flushed face before menses.

Cantharis.—Satyriasis. Priapism. Spermatorrhœa

from gonorrhœa. Severe and painful erections. Erections continuous without sensation. Violent sexual desire and continuous erection. Urethral irritation and frequent desire to urinate.

Capsicum.—Violent erections occurring only during the day, relieved only by the application of cold water. Violent erection in the morning. Trembling of the whole body during sexual excitement. Loss of sexual power and coldness of the genitals. Very sensitive to cold air. Cold chills down the back.

Carbo Veg.—Frequent nocturnal pollutions followed by depression of the nervous system.

China.—Spermatorrhœa. Pollutions. Morbid excitability of the organs. Emission induced by slight abdominal irritation. Frequent seminal emissions, ejaculations easy, followed by great weakness. Nocturnal emissions which are followed by great weakness.

Cobalt.—Seminal emissions, voluntary or involuntary, followed by pain in the lumbar region, worse on sitting.

Cocculus Ind.—Pollutions. Seminal emissions at night, with great prostration. Sadness aggravated by deep thought. Headache as if intoxicated. Imaginary fears.

Conium Mac.—Impotence. Sterility. Sexual organs very irritable. Seminal weakness with erethism and easy emission. Flaccidity of the parts with weakness of the spine and back. Emissions without erections. Hypochondriacal, morose, avoids society; sad, anxious, low-spirited from denial of carnal desires.

Cuprum Met.—Spermatorrhœa followed by epilepsy.

Digitalin.—Spermatorrhœa. Involuntary seminal emissions without dreams followed by great prostration, sadness and utter despair, with palpitation of the heart. Digitalin acts best when given in the morning.

Dioscorea.—Pollutions, two or three during the night, with dreams, pain and spasm of spermatic cord. Great weakness of the organs. Patient complains of weakness, especially about the knees. Sexual organs relaxed and cold.

Ferrum Brom. — Spermatorrhœa, with anæmia, great debility and depression of spirits. *Ferrum Mur. Tinct.*—if appetite is impaired. Anæmia following seminal discharge, in anæmic patients from over-indulgence.

Gelsemium. — Impotence. Spermatorrhœa. Organs relaxed and cold. Involuntary nocturnal emissions. Weakness and irritability of the seminal vesicles, from masturbation. Pollutions, followed next day by languor, irritability and pain referred to the occipital region, accompanied by vertigo.

Graphites.—Sterility. Satyriasis. No ejaculation follows coitus, in spite of every exertion. Sexual thoughts fill the mind to the exclusion of all others. Increase in sexual desire. Too early emission. Fear of insanity. Voluptuous irritability of the genitals.

Hamamelis.—Impotence. Organs relaxed and constantly perspire. Depressed and despondent after emission, with lascivious dreams.

Hyoscyamus.—Nymphomania, with tendency to expose the person. Sexual lust, without excitement of the fancy.

Hypericum.—Impotence from injury to spine.

Ignatia.—Impotence, with sexual desire. Amorous fancies and dreams. Impotence from grief and nervousness. Complete loss of sexual desire, with sighing. Dejected and low spirited.

Iodum.—Sterility. Impotence from atrophy of testes.

Kali Brom.—Impotence. Pollutions. Satyriasis. Loss of sexual power, with wasting of the organs, nightly emissions and great nervous irritability. Erections are normal, but persistent. Nocturnal emissions. Nervous condition from continence. Great nervous excitability. Large doses, fifteen to twenty grains three times daily, will check abnormal sexual excitement and nocturnal seminal emissions by subduing the condition of plethora. It diminishes sexual feeling and the power of erection.

Kali Iod.—Sterility from specific disease.

Lycopodium.—Impotence, erections imperfect or absent. Genital organs cold. Exciting thoughts cause no erection, though the desire is present.

Natrum Mur. — Pollutions. Spermatorrhœa. Nocturnal emissions, followed by great weakness and debility. Seminal emissions, even after coitus. Lascivious dreams and emissions, followed by back-ache, weakness of the legs, night sweats and melancholia. Erections during coitus are imperfect; the seminal discharge is small or absent. During carnal fancies, emission without erection.

Natrum Phos.—Pollutions nightly, without sensation. Erethism and lascivious dreams. Weakness of the back; trembling of the knees as if they would give way.

Nux Vomica.—Masturbation. Bad effects of pollutions. Spermatorrhœa. Impotence. Emissions towards morning followed by headache, pain in the lumbar region and weariness in the limbs. Satyriasis in alcoholics. Nervous depression, irritability, lassitude and gastric disturbances.

Phosphorus.—Satyriasis. Nymphomania. Impotence. Spermatorrhœa. Uncontrollable sexual desire in both sexes. Impotence from over-excitement of the sexual functions. When impotence follows chastity or over-indulgence Phosphorus is the remedy. Frequent emissions with great feebleness, loss of strength and flesh. Weakness in the back and limbs. Imperfect co-ordination. Sexual mania; is in constant torment for an embrace, followed by impotence. Discharge of prostatic fluid during stool. Nightly emissions with great prostration. Burning and aching in the lumbar region. Paralysis.

Platina.—Spermatorrhœa. Nymphomania. Satyriasis. Priapism. Bad effects of masturbation. Skin yellow, eyes hollow, pale and swollen; melancholy, sheepish look, epileptiform spasms. Excessive sensitiveness of the female parts, vaginismus. Voluptuous itching of the genitals. Everything around looks small, objects appear strange. Dread of death, which they apprehend to be near at hand.

Selenium.—Spermatorrhœa. Impotence. Pollutions. Nocturnal and diurnal emissions, voluntary or involuntary. Constant dribbling away of spermatic fluid, especially at stool, during micturition and when asleep. Coldness and relaxation of the sexual organs. Irritability, headache, mental confusion and sleeplessness. Paralytic weakness of the spine.

Sepia.—Pollutions, or coitus is followed by anxiety and restlessness. Seminal weakness.

Staphisagria.—Spermatorrhœa. Masturbation. Hypochondriasis from sexual excesses or perverted mental sexualities. Apathetic, gloomy, avoiding the company of the opposite sex. Irritability of the prostatic urethra. Prefers solitude, face pale, dark rings around the eyes, peevish, great emaciation; imaginary fears; anxiety; deficiency of animal heat; eyes lustreless, hair thin and dry.

Stillingia.—Spermatorrhœa from masturbation. Mental depression in alcoholics.

Stramonium.—Nymphomania, especially before menstruation; the patients become lewd in speech, thought and action and violent in manner. Strong odor of body. High degree of congestion.

Sulphur.—Masturbation. Excessive venery. Spermatorrhœa. Bad results from sexual excesses. Frequent nightly involuntary emissions, seminal fluid watery. Sexual organs relaxed and cold. Testes hang low and relaxed, erection very infrequent. Pain in back; weariness of limbs; low-spirited; debilitated; faintness; cold feet; heat on vertex. Hypochondriasis.

Ustilago Maidis.—Pollutions with erotic dreams. Pain in lumbar region; prostration and despondency. Irritability. Erotic ideas with seminal discharge.

Zincum.—Spermatorrhœa. Local irritation of the parts. Testes retracted; face pale, sunken, with deep rings around the eyes. Prolonged masturbation. Handling of the genitals. Hypochondriasis.

CHANCROIDS.

CHAPTER XVIII.

SOFT CHANCRE.

This is a contagious, virulent ulcer, usually found on the genitals of those unclean by nature and habits. Statistics show that they are frequently met with in dispensaries and hospitals, and less so in general practice. They are both hetro- and auto-inoculable; crop after crop of chancroids have been developed upon the same individual. A chancroid does not give immunity from future infection.

It is never followed by constitutional disturbances, though there is a tendency to the development of virulent bubo, which complication occurs in about one-third of all cases.

Etiology.—Chancroid can only result from the direct application, accidental or premeditated, of chancroidal pus to the skin or abraded mucous membrane, one pus corpuscle being sufficient to give rise to the characteristic lesion. It cannot be produced by syphilitic virus, by poisons of any kind, or the germs or pus of any other disease. Filthy habits, however, greatly facilitate the spread of this disgusting disease.

When the chancroidal pus is allowed to remain on or behind the glans penis and is covered by the prepuce it will, by its corroding action and maceration, eat its way through the mucous membrane destroying the epithelium and opening new points of infection which could have been prevented by cleanliness.

It is sometimes deposited upon the vaginal mucous

membrane, and after a short time by coitus conveyed to a third party who develops the chancroid while the woman escapes infection.

It may be produced by auto-inoculation, numerous ulcers resulting either from invasion of the surrounding tissue or from contact with fissures or abrasions. Infection can be carried by the finger to various parts on one's own body or conveyed to others.

Chancroids appear upon any part of the body, the head not excepted as was formerly taught; but on the head and face they run a rapid course, and are never well developed. Animals have been successfully inoculated and the true chancroid developed, but their course is comparatively mild, the ulcer being small and healing quickly. It cannot originate from syphilitic inoculation, and is never the cause of a syphilitic infection unless it acts as the point of entrance for true specific virus, producing what is known as a mixed chancre.

Clinical History.—There is no period of incubation, as infection takes place at once. In two or three, sometimes not until seven or eight days after intercourse, a well developed chancroid will appear. It commences as a small pustule or ulcer and remains an ulcer until cured. They are usually round or oval in contour, and may follow the fissures or abrasions of the skin, sometimes they are confluent. Whenever chancroidal virus is deposited upon a large abraded or granulating surface, it will be noticed that the lesion starts as a number of small ulcers from different points, which gradually enlarge and coalesce, giving a scalloped margin to the edge of the confluent chancroid. They may become serpiginous, eating irregularly into the surrounding tissue by both superficial and deep erosion. The connective tissue is especially liable to the destructive action in chancroids.

Chancroids vary greatly in size, they are usually from $\frac{1}{4}$ to $\frac{3}{4}$ of an inch in diameter. The edges are sharp and perpendicular as if punched out, though frequently they are everted from the undermining of the integument, the connective and muscular tissues being more easily destroyed than the cutaneous. The base of the ulcer is worm-eaten and irregular, yellow, tawny and sometimes red in color, covered with an adherent discharge and bleeding slightly on its removal. The discharge is profuse, yellow, creamy, greenish and sometimes bloody. The infecting quality of the pus remains until the chancroidal ulcer is cured or robbed of its virulence by complete gangrene or artificial destruction by the stronger acids, which transform the chancroid into a healthy granulating surface.

Old chancroidal conditions, however, upon the genitals and around the anus of prostitutes, which have existed for years, in time lose their virulent property.

If the ulcer has not been irritated by improper dressings it will be found to rest upon a soft, slightly inflamed base. If there has been iritation, which is usually the case, the area of imflammatory infiltration will be more prominent, and appears as an areola, which shades off into the surrounding healthy tissue. This inflammatory infiltration can easily be distinguished from the hard, firm, parchment-like feel of the true chancre, which has a sharply-defined border of induration. The chancroidal ulcer, when taken between the thumb and finger, will be found soft and pliable, unless the inflammatory exudation has been considerable, when it will feel doughy and inelastic. Chancroids are painless unless irritated. The parts, however, become irritated from uncleanliness, their anatomical location and contact with the urine, and are consequently very painful.

If the diagnosis is doubtful and the ulcerating surface cannot be exposed on account of inflammatory phimosis or when the ulcer is situated deep in the urethra, it can usually be cleared by auto-inoculation, which is performed in the following manner: A point on the chest just below the nipple, near the insertion of the Deltoid, or the outer surface of the thigh should be chosen, such selection being made on account of the small liability to produce bubonic complications. The point below the nipple should always have the preference when the ulcer shows evidence of phagedæna, experiments having demonstrated this locality to be the least likely to become phagedænic after chancroidal vaccination. The point of inoculation having been selected, some of the suspected pus is placed upon the tip of a perfectly aseptic bistoury; this is held at right angles to the body and the point introduced just through the skin, turned half way around and back again and the surplus smeared over the wound. If the pus is chancroidal in character, in from twelve to twenty-four hours after inoculation a reddish blush of commencing inflammation, accompanied by a slight burning and biting, will be noticed at its point of entrance; by the end of forty-eight hours a small pustule, surrounded by an areola of inflammatory exudation, will be developed. If this pustule be ruptured a minute chancroid ulcer, with sharp-cut edges, cup-like depression and worm-eaten base, covered with pus, will be exposed. If it remains unruptured, the pustule will in a few days dry upon the surface, the pus accumulating beneath will increase, and ulceration of the tissue will extend, constituting an ecthymatous chancroid.

When these small chancroids have served their diagnostic purpose they can easily be transformed into a simple ulcer by the application of a drop of Nitric acid and treated as such when the eschar produced by the acid becomes detached.

Chancroids may be situated on any part of the body, but are rarely found except upon or around the genitals; they are located at points most liable to abrasions or injury during coitus. In the male they are frequently found behind the corona glandis, and are usually multiple from auto-inoculation. The same can be said of the surface of the prepuce. They often occur upon the frænum and in the sulcus on either side. When the ulcer commences on the free edge of the frænum it tends to spread to the glans; when it occurs in the sulcus it usually starts at one side and rapidly eats through and destroys the frænum, sometimes opening up the frænal artery and giving rise to much hæmorrhage.

Chancroid at the meatus may be located on the commissure, on either side, or may surround it; when this occurs it leaves, on healing, an open and distended meatus. When the chancroid is situated on the glans there is usually a corresponding one on the inner surface of the prepuce covering it. When it is of the phagedænic variety it may sometimes eat into the urethra, especially if it is hidden from view by congenital or inflammatory phimosis.

Urethral chancroids are usually located in the canal a short distance from the meatus. If deep-seated they may be recognized by the local inflammatory swelling, pain, discharge, etc. In the female they are usually located on the inner surface of the labiæ, at the entrance of the vagina or on the fossa navicularis, rarely in the vagina, though occasionally on the vaginal portion of the uterus. Chancroid of the anus and rectum may occur in the female from anatomical location, but in the male it is considered an evidence of sodomy.

Chancroids are usually followed by the involvement of the nearest group of lymphatic glands. Statistics show that in about two-thirds of all cases treated these glands become inflamed, and may break down discharging a pus which has all the characteristics of that derived from a true chancroidal ulcer.

The active period of an ordinary chancroid when unirritated is about four or five weeks, when it commences to lose its virulence. This is recognized by the discharge becoming yellow and more profuse, granulations springing up and the ulcerated surface healing from the circumference to the centre, leaving a whitish scar which persists or after a time may fade gradually and disappear.

In addition to the simple chancroidal condition there are developed, clinically speaking, either from individuality, mode of life, or the location of the chancroid, certain forms which require special consideration; not that the character of the virus is dissimilar, but its results are different.

GANGRENOUS AND PHAGEDÆNIC CHANCROIDS depend upon individuality, a broken-down constitution, excessive drinking, old age, mercurial poisoning, and from certain local applications, $i.\ e.$, mercurial and other salves containing fats. Fortunately, from the better understanding of the disease and its treatment, these forms are now rare.

Gangrenous Chancroid may be engrafted upon any chancroidal condition and is recognized by increased pain, which is often excruciating, the discharge lessens and becomes sanious, the areola of inflammation extends and the ulcer becomes dry and covered with a thick, greenish, black or dry scab, which at first is firmly adherent. Suppuration soon commences, leaving, if the process has been complete and the granulating surface has not been re-infected, a simple, ulcerating wound. When re-infection has taken place the process will be again repeated. This form sometimes leads to great destruction of the surrounding tissue, and death from hæmorrhage, exhaustion, or other complications may occur. It is accompanied by marked constitutional disturbances.

Phagedæna or chronic gangrene, sometimes spoken of as serpiginous chancroid, progresses slowly and often continues for months or years. It is not accompanied by the marked local or constitutional symptoms of acute gangrene.

The phagedænic chancroid spreads slowly, eroding superficially through the connective tissue and dissecting out the blood-vessels and tendons. Sometimes it travels a great distance upon the abdomen and down the thighs; it may extend in one direction and heal in another. It may commence at the prepuce and dissect up the skin of the penis, exposing not only the penis itself but the testes as well. It may exhaust itself and finally heal without treatment, leaving much cicatrical tissue and consequent deformity of the parts.

Diphtheritic Chancroid.—This name has been given to a variety when there is little or no inflammatory action. It is painless, and is covered with firmly adherent, yellowish-white membrane, accompanied by a thin, acrid discharge. It remains active for weeks, when, without apparent cause, the membrane exfoliates and leaves behind a simple ulcer, which heals rapidly.

Follicular Chancroid, so called, results from the introduction of the infecting virus into a follicle. The venereal ulcer starts with the appearance of an acne, soon becomes inflamed and ruptures, leaving the characteristic deep chancroidal ulcer.

Treatment.—This may be prophylactic, abortive, symptomatic or remedial.

Prophylactic treatment is of no avail when the characteristic lesion has already appeared, but to the physician who finds an overlooked abrasion on his hand or who has in some way punctured his skin while making a chancroidal examination it is of the utmost importance.

The parts should be thoroughly washed with hot water or a mild antiseptic solution, then cauterized with Carbolic or Chromic acid, or Nitrate of Silver. If cauterization is objectionable, and it is within six hours from the time of the supposed infection, the virus may be destroyed without injury to the epidermis by a short immersion in a concentrated solution of Citric acid, or for an hour or two in a weak solution of Sulphate of Iron or Chromate of Potash.

Abortive Treatment.—If auto-inoculation and deep infiltration of the surrounding tissues have not occurred the abortive or escharotic treatment is indicated, imitating nature by producing a complete destruction of the diseased part; but if this treatment is imperfectly applied or some small point of infection is overlooked, the second state of the patient becomes worse than the first on account of the auto-inoculation of the increased denuded surface. Nitric and Sulphuric acids, the Acid Nitrate of Mercury, the actual cautery and removal by the knife, are, from their easy application, the agents most frequently employed.

If the chancroid is situated on the preputial edge, at the junction of the skin and mucous membrane, and there is no further involvement, the ulcer may be cleansed with Hydrogen peroxide, touched with Carbolic acid, and a circumcision performed.

When the chancroids are small and few in number the actual cautery acts very satisfactorily; it should burn deep enough to destroy all chancroidal tissues or until the parts are black and charred, then dressed with a cold water pack until the eschar comes off, when it may be treated as a simple ulcer. Nitric acid is more frequently used and may applied as follows: The chancroid is dried with absorbent be cotton or blotting paper, then cleansed thoroughly with Hydrogen peroxide, and again dried; the parts are now held so that the cup-like depression looks upwards. This is filled with a drop or more of the acid by means of a glass rod or stick and in a few moments it will turn white. The white eschar should be allowed to overlap the original edge of the chancroid, the superabundance of the acid is then removed with absorbent cotton and a drop of Carbolic acid applied to the surface to stop the pain. The ulcer is dusted with Aristol, Europhen or Europhen-Aristol and covered with antiseptic gauze until the eschar comes off, when the dusting powder should be continued until the ulcer is healed.

Sulphuric acid acts best in the Carbo-sulphuric paste which is made by mixing Sulphuric acid with willow charcoal. It is applied to the dried chancroid and pressed well down into the irregularities of the surface, where it remains as a dry black crust which peels off after a few days leaving a healthy granulating surface which sometimes heals entirely underneath the crust.

To prevent pain apply a 4 per cent. solution of Cocaine a few minutes before this treatment.

Symptomatic Treatment.—When the surface involved is large or there is evidence that a healthy reaction is about to commence cauterization is contra-indicated and other measures must be adopted. Iodoform is one of the most successful applications in this connection, the only objection being its odor. It can be best applied in the form of a paste, or it may be replaced by Aristol, Europhen, or Europhen-Aristol; these antiseptic dressings are indicated at any and all times, chancroids healing kindly from their application. Calomel, Oxide of Zinc and Bismuth sub-nitrate have also been used with benefit. Pyrogallic acid either as a powder (20 parts to 80 of starch), or as a paste, in a 5 per cent. mixture, acts well; it does not attack the healthy skin, but stimulates the chancroidal ulcer and will in time transform it into a healthy granulating surface. It should be applied night and morning and covered with gutta percha tissue and its application continued until the granulations fill up the ulcer, after which Oxide of Zinc or Calomel should be substituted to complete the healing process. Cleanliness is always of the utmost importance.

Rectal and vaginal chancroids are treated by packing with Iodoform gauze. When located at the meatus urinarius do not cauterize but apply a paste of Iodoform or Aristol pressed well into the parts or plug the meatus with a strip of Iodoform gauze. In sub-preputial chancroids inject every two or three hours, by means of a flat-nozzled syringe, first warm water and salt, then either a solution of Permanganate of Potash, 1 to 10 grains to the ounce of water, Nitrate of Silver, 5 to 15 grains to the ounce of water, or a mixture of Iodoform and Balsam of Peru. If the discharge becomes offensive it indicates a gangrenous tendency, and the glans penis must at once be exposed by slitting up the prepuce and the proper treatment followed.

When chancroids of the sub-preputial sac have eatne their way through the frænum it should be ligated and the ligature allowed to cut its way through, or it may be cut and the ends cauterized with a hot iron. A more scientific treatment is to use a pair of scissors whose edges have been rounded, one blade being passed under the band and the other heated to a white heat in the flame of an alcohol lamp, then slowly pressed together, dividing and cauterizing at the same time; this also prevents further infection.

Gangrenous Chancroids require little or no attention until the slough comes off. This may be hastened by the application of a charcoal poultice or by fomentations of a weak solution of Permanganate of Potash.

In the phagedænic variety active treatment is required. Excellent results are obtained from the Pyrogallic acid or the Carbo-sulphuric paste, the application every few days of pure Carbolic acid, or Camphor and Iodoform dressings. In some cases it will be necessary to employ the actual cautery, or to curette all the parts, remove the glans and open up sinuses, finally applying Nitric acid to the exposed surface. In every case the system must be built up by good substantial food, fresh air, etc.

Remedies, as indicated by the individuality of the case. Mercurius sol. will be indicated in simple chancroids with dirty lardaceous base. Cures have been reported made with Nitric acid and Jacaranda without local treatment. Complications will call for Arsenicum, Thuja, Sulphur, Lachesis, Hepar sulph. c., Hekla lava and Silicea.

For Special Therapy see pages 26–33.

BUBO.

CHAPTER XIX.

BUBO.

This term is now used to signify all inflamed lymphatic glands. Those connected with genito-urinary and syphilitic diseases are divided into three classes: the simple or inflammatory, the virulent and syphilitic. They occur most frequently in the inguinal region, but their situation will depend upon the location of the original point of disease. In the secondary stage of syphilis the glands throughout the body are to a certain extent involved. The simple or virulent bubo will usually be found on the side of the body on which the original point of irritation occurs and is located in the first gland or series of glands connected with it by the lymphatics. It may occur on the opposite side from lymphatic anastomosis and the buboes are sometimes bi-lateral, but only that gland or cluster of glands connected with the lesion will be involved, the general glandular system remaining unaffected.

Simple or Inflammatory Bubo is caused by straining, overlifting, horseback riding, jumping, local inflammatory disease of the uterus, rectum, urethra, etc., also by herpes, balano-posthitis, chancre, chancroid, and sometimes from undiscoverable causes.

Clinical History.—They are usually situated in the groin and vary greatly in severity, depending upon the cause and its duration. The attention is usually drawn to the parts by an uneasiness or pain on walking and possibly a sensation of fullness in the inguinal region. The glands may be slightly swollen and painful, resembling somewhat an olive with its long axis corresponding to the fold of the groin.

The inflammation may subside rapidly, or the pain and swelling increase and locomotion becomes more difficult. The glands lose their outline as the surrounding connective tissue becomes involved.

There is local swelling accompanied by a dull, heavy pain, which is sometimes sharp and spasmodic, with fever, restlessness, disturbed sleep, etc. At this time, which is generally about ten days from the commencement of the bubo, the pain and swelling may subside and the gland slowly return to its normal condition or the disease increases and suppuration take place, which is announced by chill, fever, sweat, etc. The swelling now becomes boggy, and at one point the skin appears dusky; fluctuation will be present, and by pressing into the mass the indurated walls of the abscess can easily be located. The point of softening may be at the centre or on one side of the swelling; if opened at this time probably an ounce of pus will be evacuated, but if left to itself the abscess will increase in size and after some time open at one or more points, discharging a teacupful or more of pus, or it may burrow extensively into the surrounding tissue.

The simple bubo, after opening, usually fills up with granulations and heals rapidly, but sometimes in brokendown constitutions or strumous patients the process of healing requires many months.

A subacute variety is sometimes met with where a number of glands and the tissue surrounding them are involved. It is characterized by the slow development of the bubo; suppuration is rare, and pain and swelling are not especially marked. The skin covering the glands is of a dusky hue due to the sluggish circulation. The connective tissue surrounding the glands is involved and may break down producing a peri-adenoid abscess. This suppuration frequently occurs some time in advance of degenerative changes in the glands themselves.

Virulent Bubo occurs only as the result of chancroidal infection of the involved gland. There can be no other cause and one gland only, as a rule, is involved, the lymphatics leading to it having conveyed some of the virus from the chancroid to the gland. When infection has occurred the formation of an abscess and ulceration becomes inevitable. In the early stages it is impossible to distinguish it from a simple bubo, but a virulent bubo may be suspected when its development is rapid and when it occurs during or after chancroidal infection. Statistics show that one-half of all suppurating buboes are virulent in character. In double bubo of the inguinal region one may be simple and the other virulent.

When the abscess opens, auto-inoculation will decide whether the bubo is simple or virulent. The pus from a virulent bubo has all the properties of chancroidal pus, but it is not always necessary to wait for this test, as the edges of the bubo at once assume the characteristic chancroidal appearance and the bubo itself resembes a large chancroid with everted edges and worm-eaten and uneven base, discharging a watery, yellowish or bloody pus. Unless cleanliness is maintained the surrounding parts may become infected be auto-inoculation. Many of these cases heal kindly in a few weeks while others become phagedænic and take years to cure, causing much destruction of tissue and consequent deformity. Sometimes large vessels may be dissected out and even opened, leading to fatal results.

Syphilitic Buboes always accompany hard chancre. The early glandular enlargement on the side of the original chancre may be somewhat greater han on the opposite side. The gland nearest the chancre becomes indurated a little in advance of the others, usually within ten days from the commencement of the original lesion. They are not painful, do not increase in size to any great extent and are freely movable; they rarely suppurate and may remain indurated for two or three months to several years or until all trace of the disease has been eradicated from the system. The lymphatics on the dorsum of the penis which lead to the glands will feel hard and tense, resembling cords beneath the skin. They are not painful and are often overlooked. The treatment will be that indicated for the original lesion.

Treatment.—This varies with the original cause and period of development. About one-half of all the cases of bubo, even when occurring with chancroid, are of simple inflammatory nature and under proper treatment, if commenced sufficiently early, can be aborted. The virulent bubo, however, will run its regular course, though much can be done to shorten it.

When suffering with gonorrhœa, chancroid and other troubles, which are liable to cause buboes, physical exercise must be limited and only taken in moderation; all discharges must be removed as fast as they accumulate and special attention paid to cleanliness. Irritating ointments and injections should not be used. There is much controversy as to whether the cauterization of chancroids has any detrimental effect if thoroughly applied, but there is no question as to the harm resulting from *imperfect* cauterization.

When the inflammation has commenced, rest in bed with cold applications to the parts are of the utmost importance. Cold is best employed by means of a rubber bag filled with ice water. Hot fomentations containing Aconite and Belladonna or hot poultices may be used to advantage. Many treat this condition solely by pressure; a bag partly filled with small shot or sand, or a sponge is bandaged over the part and kept moistened, thus securing continuous compression. When it is impossible to keep the patient in bed, from business or other reasons, the parts may be painted with Collodion, which contracts and thus causes pressure. These measures with the administration of Aconite, Belladonna,

Apis, Mercurius bin-iodide, Nitric acid or Hepar sulph. will usually be successful, but if after a few days resolution does not take place the bubo, be it simple or virulent, may be enucleated and the wound sutured and made to heal by first intention.

The application of Iodine is now rarely recommended on account of the complications which are likely to follow its use.

When suppuration is established, wash the parts with soap and water, then with Ether, and finally with a solution of Bichloride of Mercury, 1 to 1000. The pus can then be evacuated with the aspirator and the walls allowed to collapse when adhesion will result, unless there is a periadenoid distention of the tissues.

A small narrow-bladed bistoury may be used, making a simple incision, which is not painful if the point of entrance is first painted with a little Carbolic acid. The pus is then pressed out and the wound irrigated with a Bichloride of Mercury solution, 1 to 1000, and immediately filled to distention with warm Iodoform ointment (10 parts of Iodoform to 90 of Vaseline, not warm enough, however, to liberate the Iodine), which is introduced by a conical-pointed glass syringe. A cold compress of the Bichloride solution is then applied, covered with absorbent cotton and held in place by a T bandage.

The bubo can be opened in the manner already described and a piece of Carbolized or Iodoform gauze introduced through the incision and the pus allowed to drain away slowly. If in a day or two after evacuating the abscess the skin over the bubonic cavity drops in and becomes discolored and shrivelled, it should be removed with curved scissors and the wound treated as a simple ulcer or chancroid, as the case may require.

Sometimes a gland is left at the bottom of the bubonic ulcer and acts as a foreign body, preventing healing and keeping up this discharge. This must be removed either by ligation, cut out with curved scissors or curetted. Virulent buboes require thorough cleansing with Hydrogen peroxide and cauterization with Carbolic acid. If there is phagedæna it must be treated in the manner prescribed for that condition elsewhere. The diet should be nourishing and the indicated remedy administered.

CHAPTER XX.

SPECIAL THERAPY FOR BUBO.

Acid. Nitric.—Acts well after Mercurius or when it has failed and ulceration occurs. Ulcers remaining from the bubonic degeneration look worm-eaten are painful and tend to spread and have everted, indurated edges. The granulations bleed easily. In strumous and broken-down constitutions.

Acid. Phosphoric.—Bubonic ulcers with raised edges. Granulations pale and flabby. Edges thick, rounded and indurated.

Aconite.—Acute febrile condition with local inflammation; restlessness; anxiety; strong, full, rapid pulse; much and frequent thirst.

Alumina.—Gonorrhœal bubo, accompanied by yellowish discharge from the urethra with burning and itching, especially at the meatus.

Apis.—Inguinal glands swollen, red, hot and shiny, accompanied by great pain and sensitiveness.

Arsenicum.—Phagedænic and gangrenous buboes. Granulations red and elevated. Thin, offensive and ichorous discharge. Livid, mottled appearance of the sore. Black slough. Burning pains. Margins bleed from the slightest touch.

Badiaga.—Indurated glands, uneven and hard as stones. Violent pains, like red hot needles, through the glands.

Belladonna.—Glands enlarged, congested and inflamed. Swelling and throbbing pain in the inguinal region. Deep, radiating redness of the skin, which disappears on pressure and slowly returns. Phlegmonous inflammation.

Carbo Animalis.—Hard buboes, which threaten to suppurate, or even when there is fluctuation. Bubonic ulceration, with indurated edges and ichorous discharge.

Carbo Veg.—Excessive prostration; parts livid or mottled.

Causticum.—Acrid, corroding pus. Systemic complication. Tendency to fungous growths.

Cinnabaris.—Sometimes useful when other mercurial preparations fail.

Graphites.—Glands painful, swollen and sensitive. In broken-down constitutions.

Hepar Sulph.—Buboes which do not heal. Suppuration threatened or inevitable. If given early frequently prevents the formation of the pus.

Kali Iod.—Buboes. Glands swollen and indurated. Indolent or virulent ulceration. Thin, dark, corrosive discharge. Fistulous openings with foul discharge. Lymphatic and scrofulous or old syphilitic constitutions.

Lachesis.—Glands swollen, livid or mottled. Gangrenous and phagedænic ulcers. Broad, flat ulcers. Great prostration.

Mercurius.—Inguinal glands swollen, red, inflamed, painful and sensitive. Ulceration and suppuration taking place rapidly. Mercurius bin-iodide and Mercurius corr. act best in chancroidal buboes.

Phytolacca.—Indolent bubo. Glands swollen. Inflamed ulcers with dry, lardaceous base. General weakness.

Silicea.—Buboes which suppurate and are slow to heal.

Sulphur.—Old bubonic ulceration which will not heal.

SYPHILIS.

CHAPTER XXI.

SYPHILIS.

Syphilis is a specific infectious disease, chronic in nature, varying greatly in duration and intensity according to individuality and treatment. This disease has existed from the most ancient times, as evidenced not only by ancient writings but by prehistoric bones, which bear unmistakable evidences of syphilitic involvement. The disease was most marked and virulent in its ravages towards the end of the XV century; at that time it was called the American disease, as it was then believed to have been introduced into Europe by the sailors who shipped with Columbus. Investigation has, however, relieved the Columbian expedition of this odium, as the disease was quite prevalent in Spain before his departure. It was only coincident with Columbus' great discovery that it reappeared and spread through Europe, largely owing to the general ignorance of its character and treatment. To-day no nation is exempt from the dread disease and it is found in all parts of the world. It is more prevalent in warm climates, where it is virulent, while in the temperate zone it is moderate in its manifestations. All classes are subject to the disease, social position is no bar. It is more prone to exhibit marked secondary and tertiary symptoms in the intemperate and in early life, and in those of scrofulous or gouty diathesis.

Fatigue and excesses of all kinds also tend to increase its manifestations. At the present time it is rarely seen in its virulent form; whether this is due to acquired partial immunity as advocated by Esmarch, remains an open question. One attack usually affords protection for life, yet there are cases on record of second invasions, thus resembling other contagious diseases. It is now generally believed to be caused by the bacillus of Lustgarten, which looks very much like the bacillus of tuberculosis, but differs from it in having from two to four knobbed-like enlargements at the extremities sometimes being bent like the letter S. They are from two to seven thousandths of a millimetre in length and three ten-thousandths of a millimetre in width. They have been found within the round cells of the primary induration as well as in syphilitic growths and gummata.

Etiology.—The original cause is the introduction into the system of syphilitic virus either by inoculation, which results in a chancre at the identical point of entrance followed by the general constitutional symptoms, or by inheritance from father, mother or both, and manifesting itself by late symptoms only. Specific inoculation only occurs when the epidermis or the epithelium of the mucous membrane has been removed. The virus is not corrosive, and if the skin or mucous membrane is intact inoculation cannot possibly occur. Secretions from the original chancre, exudations from secondary involvements, as well as the blood of patients, have the power to cause, when they come in contact with the abraded surface of a healthy human being, all the manifestations of syphilis. Animals have not as yet been satisfactorily inoculated. Physiological secretions, however, are free from specific contamination, and vaccine virus taken from a syphilitic may be perfectly healthy, if it does not contain blood corpuscles, skin, etc., but the danger from such contamination is so great that it should never be taken from one suffering from the disease. Children have been nursed by syphilitic wet-nurses, with mucous patches on the nipple without harm to the child, but if, after a variable period, a break in the continuity of the mucous membrane or skin occurs, a chancre will appear after the proper period of incubation and will be followed by general syphilis. Time does not destroy the virulence of the poison. Chancres may appear on any part of the body, frequently upon the lips, tonsils, face, fingers, nipples and anus, but principally on or around the genitals. Infection may be either mediate or immediate, therefore its presence does not necessarily indicate immorality of the person affected. It may be transmitted by the neglect of antiseptic or aseptic precautions on the part of the surgeon, by the use of infected cups, spoons and towels, from kissing and in many ways other than by sexual congress.

Clinical History.—Writers on this subject have recognized for convenience of description three stages or periods. The primary, including the incubation and development of the chancre, with the early adenoid involvement. The secondary, general involvement of the glands, superficial lesions of the skin and mucous membranes. Exudations from primary and secondary lesions have the power to produce syphilis in those not protected by a previous attack. The tertiary stage may never develop. It appears as early as the third month, and may be more or less mixed with the secondary. The lesions of the skin and mucous membrane in this stage are characterized by being deep-seated and destructive and the internal organs are sometimes involved. The exudations do not have the power of propagating the disease in this stage.

Primary Stage.—In from two to seventy-two days after inoculation, but usually about the end of the third week following exposure, a chancre appears at the site of the original entrance of the virus. The part usually, during the period of incubation, does not present any abnormal condition, unless kept open by filth, inflammation or chancroid. When engrafted upon a chancroid or with chancroidal virus a mixed chancre is the result. When this occurs the character of the lesion during the first three weeks does not differ from the usual chancroid, but after the proper incubation it becomes indurated and assumes the characteristics of a true chancre. The early condition of the sore varies with the location, and whether the parts are irritated or inflamed. The lesions are characterized by the induration which is always present at some time or other during the primary lesion. It may last only a few days or for years, or it may commence before the chancre. The induration may feel like a thin layer of leather or parchment exactly underlying the chancre or a part of it, and possibly is only recognized when taking the parts between the thumb and finger. This form of induration is most common and remains but a short time, its edges are abrupt and do not shade off into the surrounding tissue. From this there is every degree to a hard, elastic, sharply defined induration, which may not only underlie the ulceration, but extend down into the tissues underneath, without tenderness to pressure or manipulation. These indurations are made up of small, round, oval or spindle-shaped cells, granular epithelium, the bacillus of Lustgarten, etc. The specific lesion found upon the induration varies with the anatomical location of the chancre On the skin or dry part of the mucous membrane it appears as an indurated papule, sometimes slightly elevated, and deep wine-red in color. After a few days it becomes covered with a scaly crust, which in time drops off. If exposed to moisture erosion will take place. Chancres situated on mucous membranes are usually erosions, and three-fourths of all chancres are of this variety. They are round, oval or somewhat irregular in form, the epithelium is absent, the surface is usually deep red, but may be very dark or gray, somewhat polished, possibly having a small grayish membrane adhering usually to its centre, together with a slight serous or sero-purulent exudation, but always small in quantity and never containing pus unless irritated. This erosion may cap a slight parchment induration situated on the prepuce, back of the corona, in the meatus, or a large indurated mass around and upon the lips. When the vitality of the patient is at a low ebb, and the chancre has been irritated or inflamed, ulceration will occur, developing a condition of granulation or a fully developed Hunterian chancre, its hard, woody and elastic induration extending far beyond its edge. Hunterian chancres have adherent edges, which slope down into the induration at the centre, giving a funnel-like aspect found in no other form of ulceration. The edges always slope towards the centre and are never undermined or sharp cut as in chancroid. In contour they are round or oval, the base is often grayish, discharging a sero-purulent fluid. When chancres are developed upon the mucous membrane of the urethra they are designated as urethral chancres and frequently escape recognition. The induration of the chancre may be felt somewhere, by external manipulation, along the course of the urethra associated with the characteristic specific glandular involvement; the diagnosis can be confirmed by the urethroscope. The herpetic form or chancre of Dubuc, the mucous tubercle of the skin, ulcerated fissure of the nipple occurring at the junction of the nipple and the breast, and the diphtheroid form, all deserve mention. Chancres vary from one or two lines to three-quarters of an inch in diameter. They may heal in two weeks or not until after secondary symptoms are well developed. They are free from pain unless irritated or inflamed. As a rule there is only one point of entrance of the specific virus, hence one lesion only; but they may be multiple if there were a number of abrasions present or another infection occurred before the development of the chancre, which may each follow its own course. Auto-inoculation cannot be made after secondary involvement until well into the third or tertiary stage, if ever. Chancres sometimes re-indurate and erode or ulcerate on the advent of the secondary manifestations; if the erosion or ulceration has not healed it may granulate without losing its induration, become covered with a whitish filament, and finally converted into a mucous patch, or it may become phagedænic, although this condition is rare outside of hospitals. With the development of the chancre changes take place in the glands which are in direct lymphatic communication. A number of these will be indurated, enlarged, retaining their oval form with their long axes in the line of the groin. At first the gland nearest the chancre is involved, but sometimes there is a large indurated gland, and on either side one or more small glands found in the chain of lymphatics called a "pleiad." It is usually located on the side in which the chancre is situated, it may occur on the opposite side of the body or on both sides; sometimes a number of glands may be bound together in a indurated mass. Specific buboes do not suppurate unless a simple inflammation be superadded, and when this occurs absorption frequently takes place. The lymphatics between the bubo and chancre are hard and feel like cords beneath the skin. Suppuration is rare and they, as well as the involved glands, slowly return to their normal condition. Hereditary syphilis never has any primary lesion.

TWENTY-THREE DIAGNOSTIC POINTS BETWEEN CHANCRE AND CHANCROID.

CHANCRE.	CHANCROID.
1. Character: A general blood disease. The chancre being always a constitutional symptom.	1. Local; the general system is never involved.
2. Period of incubation 10 to 72 days, usually about three weeks.	2. Develops rapidly. Ulceration commences immediately on the absorption of the virus. The ulcer may be well developed by the third day.
3. Cause: Sexual intercourse with another having primary or secondary syphilis; the accidental or premeditated introduction into .the system of the syphilitic virus through an abraded or punctured mucous membrane or skin.	3. Sexual intercourse with one suffering with chancroid. Inoculation by accident or design on any part of the body.

SYPHILIS.

4. Location: Most frequently on the genitals, but it may occur on the lips, face, tonsils, hands, rectum or any part of the body.	4. Usually on the genitals, but no part of the body is exempt.
5. Number: usually one, but they may be multiple from the same inoculation, then they are multiple from the beginning.	5. Usually multiple from its origin or from auto-inoculation; if not cauterized they may become confluent.
6. Appearance: It begins as an erosion or papule and remains an erosion; it may ulcerate if irritated or inflamed.	6. It begins as a pustule or ulcer and always remains an ulcer.
7. Form: Round, oval or irregular.	7. Round, oval or irregular, following creases in the skin, and with borders forming the segments of large circles.
8. Edges sloping from the circumference towards the centre. Edges adherent.	8. Edges sharp-cut as if punched out, everted or undermined.
9. Surface smooth and shiny, sometimes with a grayish pedicle in the centre.	9. Uneven, irregular, worm-eaten and without lustre.
10. Suppuration slight with serous or sero-sanguineous discharge, dry, scaly or scabby. Is not auto-inoculable.	10. Suppurates profusely. Pus very contagious. Moist or covered with a crust. Auto-inoculable.
11. Color: Deep wine-red, gray, black, livid.	11. Yellow, tawny, sometimes bright, appears as if covered with a false membrane.
12. Induration: May be parchment-like underlying the erosion, or a marked induration dipping deep into the tissue and possibly extending beyond the erosion or ulceration. It is elastic, woody and does not shade off into the surrounding tissues but is sharp cut and well defined.	12. No induration except from irritation or inflammation. When present it is doughy and shades off into the surrounding tissues.
13. Time: Induration may greatly outlast the chancre.	13. The induration always disappears with the ulceration.
14. Pain: Not painful.	14. Usually very painful.
15. Phagedæna: Rarely becomes phagedænic.	15. May become phagedænic.
16. Transmission: Not transmissible to animals.	16. Transmissible to animals but with difficulty.
17. Invasion: No tendency to invade neighboring parts; the sore soon becomes circumscribed.	17. Ulcers corrode, eating into the surrounding healthy tissue.
18. Bubo: Glands become indurated during the first or second week of the chancre.	18. Usually not until after the third week.
19. Number: A cluster or group of glands are involved.	19. One gland only, as a rule.
20. Frequency: Involvement of the glandular tissue always occurs.	20. Two-thirds of the cases have glandular involvement; of this number about one-half are inflammatory.
21. Suppuration: Rare.	21. Virulent bubo following chancroid always suppurates.

15

22. Time: Progresses slowly.	22. Progress rapid.
23. Prognosis: Local lesion good; circumscribed; general symptoms follow.	23. Local lesions are more serious; tendency to spread; no constitutional symptoms follow.

Treatment.—The old idea that syphilis is incurable is fallacious. The disease is as curable as any other infectious disease, provided the treatment is conscientiously carried out; if neglected it may cause a living if not an actual death. A case should not be taken without the distinct understanding that it will remain under care and observation for three years in the male and four in the female. All cases however do not require this prolonged medication, many are cured in a much shorter period, but a great deal depends upon the remedial agents administered during the first year. Some recover without any treatment and never manifest secondary or tertiary symptoms during their life time. The nature of the disease should be thoroughly explained as well as the contagious and infectious nature of the blood and the secretions from the primary and secondary lesions. Good hygienic conditions must be insisted upon. Alcohol in excess must be discontinued. If the use of tobacco, in all its forms, is not relinquished lesions of the mucous membranes of the mouth and throat will be frequent and troublesome. During the primary stage the teeth must be placed and kept in the best possible condition, as decayed and irregular teeth, by their irritation, are the cause of many local disorders. The chancre must never be cauterized, but should be dusted with Iodoform, Aristol, Europhen, Europhen-Aristol, Calomel or Subnitrate of Bismuth. Traditional medicine has proved by statistics that while Mercury given in this stage may somewhat hasten the healing of the chancre and postpone the appearance of secondary lesions, the tertiary symptoms are frequently more marked and virulent in character, hence mercurial treatment should never be commenced until secondary manifestations present themselves. There are cases when the diagnosis is positive, where it is sometimes advisable to give Mercury in some form before the secondary stage, as when a chancre appears on the hand or finger of the surgeon; on the lips, accompanied by much induration; on the penis, together with much swelling and œdema of the parts, interfering with micturition; or when it is absolutely necessary to relieve the specific nature at any cost. When, however, there is the least doubt, do not administer it until the diagnosis is clear. Chancres may require Arsenicum, Asafœtida, Corallium rubrum, Hepar sulphur, Kali bichromicum, Lycopodium, Phosphorus, Phosphoric acid, Silicea or Sulphur.

CHAPTER XXII.

SECONDARY SYPHILIS.

These lesions appear in from twelve days to six months, sometimes as late as the second year, but usually in about six weeks after the appearance of the chancre. The manifestations are greatly modified by treatment; in some cases they fail to make their appearance, even when no remedies are administered, the disease lying dormant in the system to break out as tertiary symptoms after many years of apparent health. Secondary syphilis is characterized by its prodromal period, in which anæmia, chloro-anæmia, icterus, bone-pains, general glandular involvement and fever precede the superficial cutaneous and mucous lesions which are pathognomonic of this stage. Alopecia is usually present, iritis and other.lesions of the eye are frequent, and nervous disturbances sometimes occur in those in whom the system is greatly saturated with the specific virus.

The prodromal period extends from the first appearance of the chancre until the development of the cutaneous lesions. During this period the symptoms are local, and in the early part there is no change in the general health;

but usually in from two to four weeks before the cutaneous outbreak a chloro-anæmic or icteric condition is developed, characterized by mental depression, listlessness, indifference, dyspnœa, physical weakness, sallow skin, sunken eyes, and neuralgic pains, periodic in character, in various parts of the head, back and limbs, occurring at night and disappearing in the morning; these symptoms are sometimes associated with gastric and hepatic disturbances, and possibly enlargement of the spleen. With these conditions there are changes in the blood itself, due to a diminution in the relative proportion of the red and white blood corpuscles, in which the red are diminished and the white increased in number, actual count showing a reduction in the number of the red corpuscles of from one-seventh to one-half. The cachectic condition may occur at any time and repeatedly during syphilitic involvement of the system, especially in those of strumous, gouty or broken-down constitutions, but the blood changes do not occur in the later stages of the disease. Near the end of the prodromal period the general involvement of the glandular system commences, although its full development does not occur until during the secondary stage. The extent of such involvement varies greatly; the glands may be so small as to be hardly distinguishable, or they may become from one-half to three-quarters of an inch in diameter. They are easily recognizable by the eye, retain their contour, are usually bi-lateral, may be soft or indurated and do not suppurate. They are especially noticeable along the posterior border of the sterno-cleido-mastoid muscle, and on the sub-occipital, posterior auricular, sub-maxillary and epitrochlear chain of lymphatics. It must be remembered, however, that indurated or swollen glands do not necessarily indicate syphilis, neither does their absence exclude it, but their disappearance positively indicates the decline of the disease.

SYPHILITIC FEVER.—A few days, possibly only a

few hours before the cutaneous eruption appears, there will be febrile symptoms without relation to the anæmic, icteric or cachectic condition already referred to. They may be of such slight degree as to pass unnoticed or the temperature may rise to 101°–105° F. The fever may be intermittent, remittent or continued in character, preceded by simple chilliness or a marked chill, the severity of the chill frequently indicating the extent of the cutaneous eruption. With the rise in temperature and pulse there are pains in the limbs and the back, malaise, thirst, etc., requiring Phytolacca, Baptisia, Chininum sulph. or Mercurius.

CUTANEOUS LESIONS.—They are called syphilodermata or syphilides and are of various kinds, possessing certain general characteristics, which greatly assist in their diagnosis. The absence of subjective symptoms is most pronounced. Itching, burning and pain are almost unknown; the exception being eruptions of the scalp, which sometimes itch. A slight burning or itching is often present at the outbreak of the eruption and when urticaria is associated with it, or where there has been a tendency to general prurigo or trichophytosis, the itching may continue and complicate the specific eruption.

The early syphilides tend to involve the whole body, while later they arrange themselves in clusters, circles or parts of a large circle; they are symmetrical in distribution, differing from the tertiary lesions of the skin which occur without reference to symmetry.

Multiplicity of character, while occurring in other diseases, is marked in syphilis, many varieties of syphilides presenting themselves upon the skin for consideration at the same time. On account of the rapid succession of the specific skin lesions the name is given to the one that is most pronounced. The color varies greatly with different conditions, being a combination of red, brown, purple or black, approximating the tinge of raw ham, coffee or chocolate. The deep tints are due to pigmentation and remain after the disappearance of the original lesion. In time they also disappear, leaving a silvery, lustrous scar.

The cutaneous lesions have a somewhat chronic history; they will subside after a certain time without treatment, yet the duration is greatly limited by the proper remedies.

The scales of the syphilides are not lustrous, but are gray or dark colored, small in size and few in number. There is frequently a zone or fringe surrounding the base of the papule; the crusts are green, black, yellowish or coffee-colored, forming layer upon layer which are prominent.

Roseola or Erythematous Syphilides appear in from three weeks to three or four months, but usually in about six weeks after the advent of the chancre. This eruption develops unnoticed or rapidly from a hot bath, chilling of the surface or excitement, and may be preceded by syphilitic fever. It may remain for months, but usually lasts from one to six weeks, appearing first on the chest, abdomen and sides, it sometimes covers the whole body, but is more frequently confined to the parts protected by the clothing. When the skin of the whole body is involved it resembles measles, at first it may be mottled or marbled in appearance, requiring much care to diagnosticate. The eruption consists of numerous small, flat (not elevated), irregular, crescentic, circular or oval spots, with indented edges, from one-eighth to one inch in diameter. These spots may be confluent, of a rose or salmon-red color, for the first few days disappearing on pressure but later leaving a dull red or brownish, tawny stain, and may scale a little and finally disappear. When the lesion has existed for any length of time other elementary lesions, papular or pustular in character, may be found associated with it and scattered over the body.

Papular Syphilides appear three to four months after the original lesion, usually, however, in about eight weeks, and remain from three weeks to two months, accompanying or following the erythematous form. It may be the original skin disorder. The papules may be pointed or flat and large or small.

The small pointed papules appear as firm pointed elevations from one sixty-fourth to one-third of an inch in diameter; they are of a rose-red or purplish color, and when irritated may develop a small vesicle or crust at the point. The eruption may be general, it may remain for months, and relapses are frequent.

The large pointed papules are lenticular in form, and may be located on the back, chest or shoulders; they are purplish-red in color, and at the apex a pustule is formed, which on breaking leaves a crust. It finally heals leaving no scar if not irritated.

The small flat papules scattered over various parts of the body or arranged in groups are the most characteristic. They increase in diameter but not in height, are smooth, hard, of a rose-red pink, and sometimes of a purplish color; at first they disappear on pressure, but later a discoloration remains. They may rupture or scale at the centre, the dried scales roll back giving the characteristic appearance of a collar or fringe surrounding the base of the papule; they gradually disappear leaving a tawny pigmentation which lasts for some time, but finally fades away without leaving a scar unless ulcerated from irritation. Relapses are frequent.

The large flat variety occurs on the face, forehead, neck, back and thighs; each papule is covered by a thin, yellow superficial scale like a crust, which has a raised border and depressed centre, the edge being distended by a little serum and surrounded by a red areola; the crust becomes detached, the papule gradually subsides and the areola of pigmentation disappears without leaving any scar. The serum of these papules is very liable to spread infection unless the patient gives them the proper care. When the large flat papules occur on the scalp they leave scabs on healing, and the enlargement of the post-cervical glands is well marked. It is not uncommon at this time to find lesions of the mucous membrane of the mouth and throat.

Papules also develop on the palms of the hands, especially in laborers; they look much like lichen-urticatus, but are distinguished from this by the absence of itching; they are circular, flat, slightly depressed and red in the centre, while at the edge they are apparently overlapped by white fringy scales. Frequently the palms of both hands will be symmetrically affected; they are papules which are not fully developed on account of the texture of the palms. Their presence is presumptive evidence of syphilis. The accidents of location, moisture and heat frequently transform papules into vegetations.

Pustular Syphilides, while not as frequent as the preceding skin lesion, are often associated with it. They vary from one sixty-fourth to half an inch in diameter, may be early or late in their appearance, persistent or transitory, arranged in groups or isolated and scattered over the body. They have three natural divisions: General superficial pustules, complicating erythema and papular syphilides, a pustular acne and a superficial ecthyma.

General Superficial Pustules may be abundantly scattered over the body in conjunction with the erythematous and papular syphilides, or they may appear alone on the forehead, upper lip or side of the nose, commencing as papules or erythematous spots, which soon become yellowish at the apex as pus is formed. They are small, superficial and sometimes run together; their base is not hardened; they are surrounded by a dull yellowish, brown or red collar; they dessicate rapidly, leaving a dark crust, the pustule healing beneath it, or ulceration may occur from which vegetations often spring. The site of the pustule is marked by a thin, white, round scar, somewhat depressed in the centre, which in time finally disappears.

Syphilitic Acne appears scattered over the body, especially on the face and lower extremities, the sebaceous glands are usually involved and from the apex of each there will project a hair. They do not appear before the sixth month and develop in from one to three weeks. When they appear earlier and are accompanied by iritis it indicates a severe form of syphilis. The duration of this syphilide is about two months, but it may be lengthened by successive invasions. Its base is red and surrounded by a ring of pigment, the apex becomes yellowish-green as the pustule develops and finally breaks and forms a scab, which may drop off in small flakes as the ulcer heals or it may remain for some time. As resolution takes place a depressed scar, somewhat deeply pigmented, slow in disappearing, will remain to mark the point of the lesion.

Superficial Ecthyma, when developed early in the second stage indicates a grave if not malignant form of syphilis; it usually appears late in the secondary stage and might be considered tertiary in character. It appears on all parts of the body, beginning as a reddened papule or erythematous patch with little or no pain, from which a broad pustule, from one-fourth to one inch in diameter, is soon formed. The pustule may become umbilicated; the base, as a rule, is not indurated, but it may be dark-red and infiltrated. The pustule dries into a thick, greenish or black scab, and ulceration may continue beneath it; when the crust is removed a quantity of thick and often bloody pus will be found. As the ecthyma develops it becomes surrounded with a dark-red or copper-colored areola, and on healing leaves a dark copper or purple-colored cicatrix, somewhat depressed and thickened, which in time gradually whitens from the centre towards the circumference.

Pigmentary Syphilides sometimes appear in patches on the side of the neck, face and chest, varying from one to two inches in diameter. They often coalesce, and the skin between the patches of pigmentation appers whiter than normal.

Vesicular Syphilides appear late in the secondary stage and are not of frequent occurrence. The base present a livid appearance which shades off into a bronzed areola. They vary in size, are usually small and pointed, and if large may be umbilicated; they may dessicate or become pustular and in maturing leave a livid spot, which remains for some time and may whiten and finally disappear.

Bulbous Syphilides appear late in the secondary stage of acquired syphilis, but are more common in the hereditary syphilis of infants. They vary from one-half to two inches in diameter, appearing isolated or scattered over the body.

The Tubercular Syphilide is a late secondary manifestation, rarely occurring before a full year after the chancre; it may develop in circular groups or be generally distributed over the body.

General Tubercules appear scattered over various parts of the body, especially on the face and forehead. They vary from a quarter to three-quarters of an inch in diameter, are round or oval in contour, somewhat elevated, and are red or copper-colored. After a short time they become covered with a scaly top that gradually falls off; the tubercule is gradually absorbed leaving a slightly brownish stain.

The Circular Groups.—These tubercles are smaller in size than the general tubercles and are always arranged in circles or segments of circles, enclosing healthy integument. They are frequently located on the face or forehead, and may last for years and on healing leave a white, smooth scab, or a slight discoloration of the skin. Sometimes new tubercules develop and form an areola around the scaly patch, producing a so-called tuberculo-squamous syphilide.

Squamous Syphilides.—Specific diseases have a tendency to scale at some period of their existence, this may be so marked that it is impossible to state for which lesion the disease should be named. This lesion rarely appears before the end of the sixth month, if earlier it is generally an accompaniment of a papular or erythematous eruption. This syphilide is a late manifestation of the second stage. They vary from one-third to one inch in diameter and are arranged in circular form, the base is slightly elevated, bluish or red in color, covered with a thin coating of scales which are small and do not overlap one another; when desquamation occurs these will be followed by other scales, but smaller. They may be located on all parts of the body, more especially on the trunks, extremities and face; on healing they leave no scar but may last for weeks or months. When located on the palmar surface they may cover large areas and often persist for some time; their base is livid, sometimes fissured, and covered with gray scales surrounded by a red collar.

Treatment of Syphilides.—The general hygiene of the skin should be the same as in non-specific cutaneous diseases. Alkaline and sulphur baths are useful and often necessary. Inunctions of Ungt. Hydrargyrum are applied to the skin in the various syphilides with the best results. When syphilides of the hands and feet become troublesome they should be immersed for a few minutes in a hot alkaline solution or scrubbed with green soap and hot water before the application of Mercurial ointment. When circumscribed, the lesions can be painted with a solution of Bichloride of Mercury, one to four grains to the ounce of Collodion. Crusts should always be removed, and the surface cleansed antiseptically and then dusted with Iodoform, Aristol, Europhen, Europhen-Aristol, Dermatol, Calomel or Sub-nitrate of Bismuth. If large surfaces are involved Iodoform must be mixed with Sub-nitrate of Bismuth or Lycopodium. When there is itching or irritation a Tar ointment can be used to advantage. If a soothing application is necessary there is none better than Ungt. Diachyli.

Remedies.— Mercurius, Graphites, Hepar, Kali iod., Acid. Nitric and Cinnabaris.

CHAPTER XXIII.

ALOPECIA.

Alopecia may occur early in the secondary stage or it may appear later in the disease, and is most marked between the third and twelfth months, attacking the hair all over the body more especially the scalp, face, eyebrows and eyelids. The hair becomes dry and lustreless, the bulbs distorted and mis-shapen; at first there is simply a general thinning of the hair, probably due to the chloro-anæmic state and fever; later the hair falls out in circular patches, varying from one-fourth to two inches in diameter.

In alopecia the scalp is smooth and appears healthy; it may be associated with papular, erythematous, pustular or vesicular lesions. The denuded spots are usually symmetrical, and show to the best advantage when the hair is cut close; in women with long hair the spots may pass unnoticed. The history will differentiate it from alopecia areata. The prognosis in the early stages of syphilis is always good, later the loss of the hair is generally permanent.

Treatment.—When no other lesions are present the scalp should be washed daily with a warm Bi-chloride of Mercury solution, 1 to 1000 or 2000, and once a week with green soap and water or with a borax solution (one egg, borax, one drachm; water, one pint;) then washed with warm water and dried. The hair must be well brushed for three minutes daily, and one of the following applications used. If dry and brittle:

℞ Flor. Sulphur, ... ʒi.
    Vaseline, ... ʒi.
    M.
Sig. Rub a little into the roots of the hair at bed-time.

If the hair is not especially brittle, one of the following can be used:

℞ Tinct. Capsicum Annuum, ... ʒii.
    Glycerin, ... ʒii.
    Aq. Colognii, ... ʒi.
    M.
Sig. A small portion to be rubbed into the bald spots at bed-time to stimulate the parts.

℞ Acid. Lactic, ... gr. viii.
    Acid. Boracic, ... ℈iiss.
    Spts. Vini Gallici, ... ʒi.
    Aqua Dest., ... ʒx.
    M.
Sig. A teaspoonful to be rubbed into the roots of the hair at bed-time.

If moist eruptions occur they should be dusted with Calomel or Ungt. Hydrargyrum ammoniatum may be used with an occasional application of a Carbolic acid solution.

Remedies.—Hepar sulphur, Carbo veg., Kali iod. and Lycopodium.

CHAPTER XXIV.

ONYCHIA AND PARONYCHIA.

Diseases of the nails and adjacent parts occur in the latter part of the secondary and during the tertiary stage; they may be mild or severe in form, of long or short duration, but many are noted for their persistency.

Onychia and paronychia are usually so intimately associated that they are best described together. Some divide the disease into two classes, calling it onychia when it begins in the nail and extends to the surrounding parts, and paronychia when it commences in the tissue around the nail. The nail loses its lustre, becomes grayish-yellow in color, dry and brittle, the surface is irregularly corrugated, with possibly here and there round spots which have become softened, disintegrated and have been removed by the general washing and friction of the hands. The nails may be separated from their attachments and the edges everted; the skin and other tissues in apposition to them at the side or base of the nail or both may be swollen, œdematous, of a purplish-red color and may contain pus, or they may be fissured and scaly. Sometimes the nail increases greatly in size, becoming three or four times its normal thickness; it may be tilted upon one side and beneath it there may extend a granulated, indolent surface which exudes a grumous fluid. Mucous patches frequently undermine the nail and may separate it completely from the underlying tissue. The nail may be thrown off, exfoliation in some cases occurring without any appreciable lesion. The infiltrated skin around the nail and ends of the fingers may continue scaly for some time, but eventually, even in the most severe cases of onychia, the digital extremities return nearly to their normal condition.

Treatment.—Pain, uneasiness and congestion of the parts will be greatly relieved by immersion for fifteen minutes, three times daily, in a solution of carbolized water (30 drops of carbolic acid to the quart of hot water), then dried and dressed with Ungt. Hydrargyrum ammoniatum, and protected by a glove finger. If cracks or fissures are present Zinc. oxid. gr. xxx, may be added to each ounce of the Mercurial salve, and the granulating and ulcerated surface should be dusted with Aristol, Europhen, Iodol, Dermatol or Iodoform. The rapid disappearance of the indurated and scaly surface will be greatly facilitated by painting it every other day with Pyrozone 25 per cent., a saturated solution of Salicylic acid and Collodion or a solution of one to four grains of Bi-chloride of Mercury to the ounce of Collodion.

Remedies.—Mercurius in its various forms, Kali iod., Graphites, Antimonium crudum and Arsenicum.

CHAPTER XXV.

LESIONS OF THE MUCOUS MEMBRANE.

These are most marked in the mouth, throat and about the anus, although any of the outlets of the body may become involved. They appear at any time during the secondary stage and are sometimes noticed during the tertiary. The original lesion may even be located on any of the mucous membranes. From three to eight weeks after the appearance of chancre an erythema, diffused or circumscribed, may appear on the mucous membrane of the mouth and throat, most frequently on the fauces. It may spread upward and involve the pharynx, to the nasal mucous membrane, eustachian tube or down the larynx and forward to the buccal cavity. It resembles a cold, with more or less aphonia, and other symptoms of irritation of the parts and the inflamed surface is dull red in color; this constitutes the sore throat of early syphilis which often escapes recognition. It may disappear in a few days or lead to ulceration, especially in those who continue to use tobacco and are careless about the care of their teeth. It occurs more frequently in the male than in the female. The ulcerations are round, oval and sometimes irregular in form; at first they are covered with a grayish-white pedicle, which on removal leaves a smooth raw surface, and when irritated the ulcers may become indurated around the edges; they are generally located upon the fauces and arch of the palate over the tonsils, sides of the tongue, inner surface of the mouth, etc.

When the irritation has caused induration the ulcerations appear deep, with sharp cut borders and outline, the base being unhealthy and tawny yellow in color. The irritated ulcerations are located most frequently at the corners of the mouth, on the tongue, tonsils and anus. Lesions of the mouth and throat are attended with some swelling of the sub-maxillary glands, sometimes with a slight swelling and soreness of the tonsils, the ulcerations usually lasting two or three weeks.

MUCOUS PATCHES develop on the mucous membrane, also upon the skin when moisture is present. They are most frequently observed in the mouth, on the soft palate, pharynx, tongue, and in the neighborhood of the anus, and may appear during the early or late stages of syphilis. These patches are rounded, oval or irregular in contour, usually somewhat elevated, and are pale or rose-colored. On the tonsils they may give rise to vegetations and ulceration. On the skin they frequently granulate, grow rapidly and proliferate, producing specific condylomata, which are found about the anus, between the scrotum and thighs, and between the toes. When mucous patches appear around the mouth and are dry they are dull red in color. They also appear in conjunction with onychia and paronychia, eating under the nails like a soft corn. A variety of mucous patches appear on the tongue, which commence as macules about the size of a millet seed, spreading over the surface or as flat circular papules of various sizes, which are scattered over the upper surface and sides accompanied by superficial or deep infiltration, or they may result from irritation from a sharp edged or necrosed tooth.

When condylomata appear around the female genitals they exude an offensive discharge. The secretions from all mucous patches are especially contagious, and patients must be warned at this time against kissing and to take special care of utensils used by themselves and others.

SCALY PATCHES are located on the dorsum or sides of the tongue, buccal mucous membrane or pharynx; they are rounded or irregular in form, flat and smooth, white or bluish-white in color, giving the appearance of having been recently touched with Nitrate of Silver. This white surface is not easily removed; the more severe the lesion the whiter will be the scales, which may crack, bleed and become painful, though pain is usually absent.

Prognosis.—Good in lesions of the mucous membranes.

Treatment.—Lesions of the mucous membrane in secondary syphilis require prophylactic, local and remedial measures. Cleanliness is of the first importance. The severity of the lesions will largely depend on the care and attention they are given; the teeth should be brushed night and morning and the mouth and throat gargled with Listerine, Tincture of Myrrh, Chlorate of Potash, Bicarbonate of Soda, Sodium chloride or Borax, diluted with warm water. Tobacco in all forms must be discarded. The treatment of these lesions must depend upon their severity. They are relieved by solutions of Borax, Sodium bicarbonate, Chlorate of Potash, Alum, Dobell's Solution, Electrozone, Listerine or Hamamelis, diluted with warm water, to suit the individual case, used as a gargle or spray, but the best results are obtained by the following prescription, recommended by Taylor:

℞ Sodium Borat., ... ℨiii.
    Tr. Catechu, ... ℨiv.
    Tr. Myrrhæ, ... ℨiv.
    Aqua, ... ℥vii.
M.

which may be used at any time. A gargle of Bichloride of Mercury, 1 to 5,000 or 10,000, is sometimes useful. Mucous patches and ulcers can be treated by applications of Nitrate of Silver, ten to twenty grains to the ounce, applied every few days, but the daily application of Glycero-iodide (ten grains of Iodine to one ounce of Glycerine gives quicker and better results). Before the application of the Nitrate of Silver or Iodine the parts must be sprayed with a cleansing solution. External mucous patches require, in addition to those already mentioned, applications of Calomel, Iodoform, Dermatol, Aristol, etc. Vegetations may be treated as directed for that condition on page 19.

Remedies.—Mercurius,* Kali bich., Acid Nitric., Phytolacca, Kali mur., Calc. fluor., Acid Fluoric., and Kali iod.

---

*If Mercury is administered in appreciable doses the closest attention must be paid to the mouth, and on the slightest evidence of mercurialization the treatment must be discontinued or modified, and a strong solution of Alum and warm water or brandy and water used three or four times daily as a mouth wash. When the mucous membrane becomes swollen and inflamed, it must be painted daily with equal parts of Tinctures of Myrrh and Iodine, and a Borax and hot water gargle used frequently. The pain of the ulcerated surfaces is greatly relieved by painting with a 4 per cent. solution of Cocaine. A hot bath should be taken at bed time, the food should be fluid and easily digested. A choice can be made of Panopepton, liquid peptonoids, sarco-peptones, milk, beef tea, mutton and clam broth, Somatose, etc., together with the administration of Chlorate of Potash internally.

CHAPTER XXVI.

CONJUNCTIVA, CORNEA AND SCLERA.

CONJUNCTIVA.—While syphilitic lesions of the conjunctiva are rare, they may occur in any stage of the disease. Conjunctival chancre is most frequently seen at the ciliary border, involving also the integument of the lid, but it may be limited to the conjunctiva, and if so is most apt to appear in the cul de sac, where it often takes the form of deep ulceration. The pre-auricular gland is enlarged and other neighboring glands may be affected. Obstinate catarrhal conjunctivitis, which may pass over into the trachomatous form, sometimes occurs as a secondary symptom, especially where iritis is present.

MUCOUS PATCHES may develop upon the ocular conjunctiva, though the cul de sac is the usual site. They appear as uneven, lardaceous ulcers with ragged edges.

GUMMY INFILTRATION of the bulbar conjunctiva appears as a livid tumor freely movable upon the subjacent tissue. The infiltration may be circumscribed or diffuse, and implication of the sclera will be indicated by the absence of mobility. The surrounding tissue is somewhat swollen and ulceration may follow in a comparatively short time, the process of repair being slow and resulting in a firm cicatrix.

CORNEA—KERATITIS PARENCHYMATOSA.

Etiology.—Nearly two-thirds of the cases of this disease are said to be due to inherited syphilis. It is especially a disease of childhood and youth, but has been seen as late as the sixtieth year. Females are more liable than males, and are apt to be attacked at an earlier age. Hutchinson's teeth are found in about one-quarter of the cases, but do not necessarily indicate syphilitic origin.

Pathology.—The disease is essentially an inflammatory infiltration of the corneal parenchyma, affecting particularly the deeper layers, often occupying the membrane throughout its extent. In severe cases, the epithelial coverings of the membranes of Bowman and Descemet may participate. The peripheral circulation is engorged and there is a formation of new vessels. The cornea is much thickened, its constituent lamellæ being swollen by the imbibition of serous effusion, and its resisting power often greatly reduced. The exudation undergoes gradual absorption, leaving the corneal tissue nearly or quite free from pathological change, or sclerosis may occur in places.

The disease may be vascular or non-vascular; cases from syphilis are said to be more apt to take the latter form.

Clinical History.—Vascular Form.—A variable degree of injection of the superficial and deep ciliary vessels precedes the formation of slight opacities at the centre or periphery of the cornea; if the latter, but one portion may be at first affected, or several foci may appear at once at different points in the circumference. The opacities gradually increase in size and encroach upon the membrane, a fine haziness occupying the space between them. Later they become confluent in places and the haziness increases until the whole cornea assumes the so-called ground-glass appearance, leaving the iris dimly visible but rendering it impossible to examine the details of the fundus. The vessels constituting the marginal loops at the corneal periphery are engorged and pass forward in the cornea for a certain distance, forming a vascular circle deep in its substance. New vessels are formed, which pass toward the centre here and there, especially following the opacity.

The so-called salmon patch of Hutchinson is due to an agglomeration of these vessels, forming a reddish blotch of considerable size, usually toward the centre of the membrane. In severe cases the vascularity may extend throughout the cornea, making it appear uniformly red, the condition differing from pannus in the fact that the vessels are within the substance of the cornea and not upon its surface, the color and appearances being altered by the intervening haziness.

At the height of the disease the epithelial covering of the membranes of Descemet and Bowman is often attacked, resulting in the former case in the so-called punctate opacities of the posterior layer, and in the latter destroying the smooth, glistening appearance of the external surface of the normal cornea, which takes on a roughened aspect.

In certain cases the cornea becomes soaked and swollen by the amount of serous effusion present, causing a degree of softening and a tendency to bulging in places, which may result later in alterations of the normal curvature and even staphyloma. Pain, photophobia and lachrymation vary widely in proportion to the vascularity, at times being almost nil, but in bad cases often very severe.

Vision is always greatly reduced. The pupil is contracted and unusually resistant to mydriatics, the swollen tissue opposing their absorption.

Iritis is a common complication and there is hyperæmia of the entire uveal tract. Choroiditis with opacities of the vitreous, and retinitis may also occur, though they will be masked for a time by the corneal haziness. In cases which have been improperly treated, especially where irritants have been used, cyclitis may develop. The disease increases with some rapidity at first, culminating in from four to six weeks, when it may be stationary for a time, after which the vascularity lessens and the other symptoms begin to abate. The cornea clears slowly, from the periphery toward the centre, where the haziness persists for a considerable period, months, sometimes years, elapsing before the process is completed. Many times when the opacity has apparently disappeared, careful examination will reveal the presence of a fine diffuse haziness materially interfering with vision.

246   SYPHILIS.

In severe cases the intensity of the inflammation may produce corneal sclerosis in spots, leaving permanent, whitish, opaque patches. The disease is essentially chronic, and almost always attacks both eyes, especially when from syphilis. The second eye is usually affected soon after the first, but may not be involved until much later.

Prognosis.—This is generally good, useful vision being finally attained, as a rule, though it may never reach normal acuity. Intra-ocular complications affect the prognosis unfavorably; where irido-cyclitis intervenes the eye may even be lost. Impaired vitality and bad surroundings reduce the chances. Relapses are frequent, both of the primary disease and complications, but recurrence is rare after complete recovery.

Non-Vascular Form.—The same conditions of the cornea present, but in a lesser degree, and usually with but little vascularity or irritation.

Subjective symptoms, with the exception of reduced vision, are apt to be trifling. The course is equally chronic, and complications are comparatively rare. The ultimate prognosis is better than in the vascular form.

Treatment.—Use of the eyes should be interdicted, and they should be protected from bright light and irritants. If iritis occur Atropine or Scopolamine should be instilled, and in severe cases this should be done as a precautionary measure. The general nutrition of the patient should be improved by all possible means. Should glaucoma supervene, Scopolamine may be tried, but unless the result is immediately favorable an iridectomy should be made. If staphyloma threaten late in the disease, a pressure bandage should be applied and a solution of Eserine, 1 to 200, instilled.

Aurum Muriat.—Hereditary syphilis, either vascular or non-vascular form. Some photophobia. Lachrymation apt to be irritating. Orbital bones sore and bruised. One of the best remedies, especially if the mental symptoms of the drug be present.

Calc. Hypophos.—Useful late in the disease if there is a tendency to staphyloma.

Kali Iod.—No special ocular symptoms; prescribed on general conditions.

Kali Mur.—Symptoms moderate and not characteristic. Valuable for absorbing infiltration and clearing up diffuse haziness.

Merc. Sol.—High grade of inflammation. Irritating lachrymation. Useful when iritis is present. Throbbing, shooting and sticking pains in and around the eye. Aggravation at night, with general symptoms of the drug.

Sulph.—Some photophobia, with feeling of sand in the eyes or stitches like needle pricks or broken glass. Especially indicated if general symptoms are present. Useful in clearing the cornea.

KERATO-MALACIA.—This rare disease may occur as a result of hereditary syphilis and is peculiar to infants and young children. It usually attacks both eyes and is essentially a necrosis of the cornea followed by purulent degeneration and rapid destruction.

Clinical History.—Dryness of the conjunctiva, especially on either side of the cornea, the spots later assuming a lardaceous appearance and extending rapidly over the entire membrane and the cornea, which becomes cloudy and anæsthetic. Necrosis begins in the centre, spreading rapidly and passing over into purulent degeneration.

Hæmorrhage into the vitreous may occur and panophthalmitis may result. Patients are generally in bad condition and may die before the termination of the ocular disease.

Prognosis is bad both for sight and life, but improves with the age of the child.

Treatment should be constitutional.

GUMMY SCLERITIS is either diffuse or circumscribed

and may begin in the sclera or extend from gumma of the ciliary body. The latter form is very intractable and apt to result in staphyloma. If the disease be confined to the sclera the prognosis is good.

Constitutional treatment is indicated.

CHAPTER XXVII.

DISEASES OF THE UVEAL TRACT.

IRITIS.—Etiology.—About one-half of all cases of iritis are due to syphilis, hereditary or acquired. In adults it results from the acquired form and the majority of cases are secondary manifestations, usually appearing after the first eruption on the skin or within a year after infection. Only ten to fifteen per cent. are of the gummous variety.

In childhood the disease should excite suspicion, as, except from traumatism, it is very rare in early life unless from hereditary syphilis, and is then most often seen about puberty and accompanying keratitis parenchymatosa; although cases occur in infancy, and occasionally, though seldom, in utero.

The disease is always plastic in character and varies greatly in severity, being at times insidious in its approach and forming adhesions at the pupillary margin with few or no symptoms. On the other hand, it may take the form of a violent irido-cyclitis; the average case, however, being of a medium degree of intensity and differing in no respect from ordinary iritis unless papules or gumma appear on the iris, these being characteristic of syphilis.

Clinical History.—There is circumcorneal injection; the iris is dull, velvety and discolored, the normal folds being lost from the swelling and infiltration. Occasionally spots of exudation or hæmorrhage appear on its surface. The pupil is contracted and motionless, the use of mydriatics revealing attachments to the lens capsule. The aqueous humor is more or less hazy, and this must be distinguished from a dull, steamy aspect of the cornea which appears in severe cases. Some photophobia and lachrymation may be present and the ball may be tender to touch to a degree dependent upon the severity of the inflammation.

There is more or less pain in and around the eye, sometimes including the entire distribution of the fifth nerve on the affected side. The pain is aggravated at night, when it may be very intense. Vision is soon reduced; in bad cases, where the entire pupillary margin is adherent, or where masses of exudation are deposited within the pupillary area, it may be nearly or quite lost.

Opacities may appear in the aqueous humor from exudative deposit, and in rare instances masses of gray, gelatinous exudation may occupy a considerable portion of the anterior chamber, sometimes resembling a luxated cataractous lens. This is usually soon absorbed. If the ciliary body be implicated there will be exquisite sensitiveness at some point, all the symptoms will be aggravated, and the veins of the iris will be dilated, with chemosis and considerable swelling of the lids.

This condition may pass over into the chronic form of irido-cyclitis, with the formation of new vessels on the surface of the iris, which may become bright yellow or green in color, finally changing to the slate-gray of atrophy, with great thinning of the membrane. Relapses are frequent.

A peculiarity of the syphilitic form of the disease is that it may be limited to a certain portion of the iris, especially when papulous or gummous, the first corresponding to the papular eruption.

Papular Form.—One to four papules are developed in the iris, varying in size from a pin head to a millet seed, usually reddish-brown in color and often with a copper colored zone at the base. These are frequently situated in the internal and inferior quadrant of the iris, either near the pupillary border or at the periphery, and may be crossed by fine vessels. The papules later undergo absorption, leaving no trace behind, differing in this respect from the

Gummous Form.—This presents yellowish or brownish nodular masses, sometimes streaked with blood, with little change in the intervening tissue. These originate deep in the connective tissue, are apt to be large, solitary and peripheral, in some cases touching the posterior wall of the cornea. Extension is toward the ciliary body, and when very large they may cause phthisis bulbi by interfering with secretion. If small and peripherally situated, the over-lapping scleral border may almost conceal them. Later fatty degeneration ensues and they are absorbed, an adherent gray cicatrix marking their site.

Syphilitic iritis may be bi-lateral, but one eye is usually attacked before the other.

Prognosis.—The prognosis is fair, some cases recovering entirely, about fifty per cent. losing half their vision, while in severe cases the eye may be totally lost.

Treatment.—The patient must keep in bed. The whole head on the affected side must be kept warm by a thick cotton pad. If pain is severe, relief may be obtained by applying a hot salt bag. In isolated cases the ice bag may prove more grateful to the patient. All adhesions should be broken down as rapidly as possible by the use of mydriatics, Atropine, in a solution of four grains to the ounce, or Scopolamine hydrobromate, Hyoscyamine hydrobromate or Duboisine sulphate, in solutions of 1 to 200. If there is any tendency to increased tension Scopolamine should be the drug chosen. Every effort should be made to fully dilate the pupil and keep it so, using the mydriatic as often as once in every two hours if necessary, but carefully watching the patient for symptoms of poisoning.

The diet should be simple and constipation should be avoided.

Asafœt.—Intermittent, throbbing, darting or lacerating pains in and around the eye, often from within outward, relieved by touch or pressure, often aggravated at night. Adapted to patients who have been overdosed with Mercury.

Aurum.—Also useful after over-dosing with Mercury and Potash. Severe boring, tearing or pressive pains in the eye and head. Bones of the orbit and skull painful as if broken, aggravated by lying down. Pain extends from above downwards and from without inwards, aggravated by rest and pressure. Vision indistinct. Especially useful if the mental symptoms of the drug are present.

Cinnabar.—Pain beginning at the inner canthus and extending along the edge of the orbit to the outer canthus; or pain may encircle the eye apparently in the rim of the orbit. Aggravation at night. Useful in the gummous form.

Clematis.—Stitches in the inner canthus of the eye. Sore smarting in the eyes; sensitive to cold air. Worse from cold bathing. Adapted to chronic forms of iritis.

Kali Iod.—When indicated by general conditions. Majority of the symptoms appear during rest and go off during motion. Aggravation at night. No special symptoms, but usually a severe form of iritis.

Merc. Corr.—Inflammation very intense. Severe pain. Boring, tearing or cutting in and around eyes and frontal region. Aggravated at night and by damp weather, with general mercurial symptoms. One of our most valuable remedies for this disease.

Merc. Dulc.—Disease presenting mercurial symptoms, but not so severe; apt to be somewhat slow. Especially useful in breaking down adhesions, and for this purpose should be given as low as the 3rd or 4th decimal, every three hours.

Merc. Proto-Iod.—With mercurial symptoms, there is the characteristic yellow base at the tongue.

Sulphur.—Fine sticking pains in the eyes as from needles or broken glass. In cases which do not seem to do well, especially if general symptoms for the drug are present. Sometimes very useful in syphilitic iritis.

Thuja. — Conjunctiva red like blood. Iritis with condylomata on the iris, large, wart-like. Sharp sticking in the eye, with much heat in and around it. Pain in left frontal eminence and in right side of the head, as if a nail were driven in. Aggravation after 3 P. M., at night, and from heat of the bed. Amelioration from warmth.

CYCLITIS.—This is rare as a primary disease, being commonly an extension of iritis or choroiditis. It may occur in two forms, the acute, with all the symptoms of an intense iritis, *great sensitiveness of the ciliary region*, chemosis and considerable swelling of the lids, or there may be gumma of the ciliary body, showing as a bluish tumor through the sclera.

In the first form we have all the symptoms of iritis much exaggerated, aqueous humor turbid, complete synechia, entire iris glued to lens capsule, veins of the iris dilated, deep anterior chamber, opacities in the anterior part of the vitreous humor, with great impairment of vision.

The gummy form may be partial, vision being badly affected. Later the gumma absorbs, leaving bluish staphyloma. Tension may be plus at first, but is apt to be minus afterwards from interference with secretion consequent upon atrophy of the affected part. If severe, atrophy of the globe may follow.

Prognosis.—This is grave.

Treatment.—Should be the same as for iritis.

IRIDO-CHOROIDITIS.—This is a rare form of disease. It may be due to the extension of a severe parenchymatous iritis, or result from gumma in the ciliary body, extending both to the iris and the choroid. It is a very rapid and violent form of disease, and except under the most careful treatment apt to end in the destruction of the eye.

Treatment is the same as for iritis and cyclitis.

CHOROIDITIS.—The majority of cases of this disease result from syphilis, usually from the acquired, sometimes from the hereditary form, and in rare cases it is congenital.

When from acquired syphilis it commonly occurs during the first two years, but may be much later. It most frequently takes the form of choroiditis disseminata, but in some cases the retina is involved, constituting choroidoretinitis.

Choroiditis Disseminata.—If the disease be acute, we find small round patches of exudation, beginning as a rule in the periphery, and appearing as yellowish, ill-defined spots. These may be on the inner surface of the choroid or in its stroma. As the exudation is absorbed its site becomes thinned and later atrophied, the sclera showing through as a white patch, which in time becomes more or less surrounded by black pigment.

At first the vitreous may be somewhat hazy and the optic disc red. As the disease progresses and encroaches further upon the fundus the spots enlarge, perhaps coalescing here and there, until, in old cases, the entire membrane may be riddled with atrophy. Frequently, however, in the syphilitic form, the patches remain small and show no tendency to coalesce; or the disease may be chronic from the beginning, the stage of exudation not being apparent, the patches of atrophy being gradually developed.

The disease may begin centrally in the fundus, and here a form often found in syphilis presents numerous small, white patches, surrounded by a reddish zone, with little tendency to coalesce or change in form.

There is no pain in the primary form of the disease. Vision varies widely according to the portion of the fundus affected. If the disease is confined to the periphery there may be little or no loss of vision. As it approaches the posterior pole, however, visual defects are markedly increased. When the macular region is invaded metamorphopsia and micropsia may be present, from compression of the retinal elements, and the sight will be very poor. When the periphery is most affected there may be marked contraction of the field, while atrophic patches in the posterior part of the fundus more frequently result in scotomata, varying in size and number.

The range of accommodation may be limited, and hemeralopia may be present.

Serious implication of the vitreous often occurs in the later stages, with numerous opacities, which still further reduce vision.

In old cases blindness often results from atrophy of the retina and optic nerve, and sometimes cataract is developed.

The course is very slow and the progress, though best in syphilitic forms, is poor, as the disease is obstinate, with great tendency to recurrence. The vitreous may clear up, especially if the opacity be diffuse, but circumscribed opacities, if large, are apt to be permanent.

When due to acquired syphilis, both eyes are usually affected.

Choroido-Retinitis.—This form of the disease occurs at the end of the secondary stage or later, and is characterized by diffuse dust-like opacities in the vitreous (best seen with the plane mirror and subdued light), and circumscribed opacity about the optic disc extending more or less on the retina along the large vessels. Later choroidal patches appear, often first in the region of the macula, afterwards more widely scattered, but usually smaller.

The disease is obstinate and shows great tendency to relapse. In the later stages there is proliferation of the pigment epithelium, which invades the retina, as is shown by its peculiar bone-corpuscle arrangement and its proximity to the retinal vessels.

The implication of the retina causes irritation of and dragging upon this membrane; as a result phosphenes are present in the earlier stages, to be succeeded later by metamorphopsia, micropsia and scotomata. The color sense is normal except in scotomata, where it is lost. Vision decreases rapidly, and hemeralopia develops late in the disease. The vitreous gradually clears up, but vision deteriorates and atrophy of the optic nerve may result.

When the bone-corpuscle arrangement is marked the disease may be mistaken for retinitis pigmentosa. The presence of the dust-like opacity of the vitreous, the fact that the patient is past middle age, the late occurrence of hemeralopia and the presence of choroidal changes constituting the differential signs.

Treatment.—The general health of the patient should be improved as far as possible, all visual labor should be prohibited and the eyes should be protected from bright light by smoked glasses. Stimulants should be forbidden.

Aurum.—Adapted to either form of the disease but in choroiditis there are usually no special indications and we must rely on general conditions in the choice of a remedy.

Kali Iod.— The best general remedy for syphilitic choroiditis of any form, especially where haziness or opacities of the vitreous are present.

Kali Mur.—Sometimes useful for the absorption of the exudation in the earlier stages.

Mercurius.—Must be selected on the general indications.

Sulphur.—Useful as an inter-current, or when apparently well indicated remedies fail of effect. May afford aid in clearing up the vitreous.

VITREOUS HUMOR.—In syphilitic affections of the ciliary body, choroid and retina, opacities of the vitreous are always present, the only form which is characteristic being that of fine dust, which appears on ordinary examination as a diffuse haziness, and is only properly recognized by the use of the plane mirror with reduced illumination.

Opacities may, however, take many forms and vary much in size. They result from an invasion of the vitreous by exudation or hæmorrhage, and appear as flakes, strings, dots or membranes, usually more or less movable; sometimes fixed. Their rapidity of motion depends upon the degree of fluidity of the vitreous, and they are largely responsible for the reduction of vision in the above mentioned diseases. A diffuse cloudiness and the smaller opacities may be entirely absorbed, but large membranes or flakes are apt to be permanent. Those caused by syphilis offer the best prognosis.

Relapses are not unusual.

Treatment should be directed to the primary disease, although the Iodide of Potash is a most excellent remedy for many of these conditions.

CHAPTER XXVIII.

DISEASES OF THE RETINA AND OPTIC NERVE.

RETINITIS.—The retina may be involved at any stage of acquired syphilis, or as a result of hereditary disease, the condition varying according to the period at which it appears. Three forms are recognized, viz: Irritation, diffuse inflammation and central recurrent retinitis.

Retinal Irritation is characterized by indistinctness of the outlines of the optic disc, which is somewhat reddened, and congestion of the retina, shown by enlargement and tortuosity of the veins, may appear soon after primary infection, subsiding later or passing over into the second form.

Diffuse Retinitis commonly occurs late in the secondary stage, may be sudden in its onset, and presents the following

Clinical History.—Enlargement and tortuosity of the retinal veins with reduction in size of the arteries; the optic disc is reddened, somewhat swollen, and its outlines are indistinct; there is serous effusion into the surrounding retina, sometimes involving the macular region, being especially prominent along the course of the vessels and gradually shading off into the normal tissue. A slight striation may be observed immediately around the disc, due to accentuation of the retinal nerve fibre layer from swelling. The serous effusion may be slight, showing only a faint grayish haze, which is best seen with weak illumination. Hæmorrhage is rare and if present is slight, the appearances being usually, not always, limited to the vicinity of the disc and macula.

The disease may be associated with choroiditis and iritis, and there may be haziness of the vitreous.

Vision is apt to be seriously affected, especially if complications be present, but it may fluctuate greatly. The affection, unless very mild, is often obstinate from its great tendency to repeated relapse, and it not uncommonly lasts for months. The inflammation is sometimes confined to one eye, but frequently its fellow participates later.

Prognosis.—This is good in the uncomplicated form of the disease, but as a rule only after long treatment, unless the case be exceptionally mild. It is less favorable when frequent relapses occur, which may induce atrophy of the optic nerve.

Central Recurrent Retinitis, the rarest form, appears late in the course of syphilitic infection and may be confined to one eye, but usually affects both.

Minute spots are seen in the macula, which are chiefly remarkable for the suddenness with which they appear and disappear, producing corresponding changes in vision, which at first may clear up completely between attacks, but later does so only partially. When the disease becomes established there is central scotoma for color, the light sense being usually preserved, the field of vision and color sense being otherwise normal.

Metamorphopsia, micropsia and hemeralopia may be present. The disease is stubborn and generally results in serious impairment of vision.

PAPILLITIS AND PAPILLO-RETINITIS occur as a result of syphilitic brain disease, either in the form of meningitis or of cerebral gumma, the infection being propagated along the lymphatic channels in the coats of the vessels. In the first form we have the usual picture of choked disc, the papilla being reddened, much swollen, and grayish as a result of infiltration; the veins are partially buried in the swollen tissue of the disc, and enlarged and tortuous beyond, the arteries being reduced in size. At the height of the disease the papilla presents the so-called "woolly" appearance, the vessels are lost in the centre and flammiform hæmorrhages are present near the margin. Later as a result of varicosity and sclerosis of the nerve fibres, the color of the disc changes and numerous striated white spots are seen. White lines appear on the sides of the vessels, extending somewhat on the retina, the result of sclerosis of their coats.

PAPILLO-RETINITIS.—Here the disease extends for a certain distance upon the retina, especially in the region of the macula. The disc is apparently less elevated because the surrounding retina participates in the swelling, which, however, in some cases may not be great. The hæmorrhages spread more upon the retina and may encircle the disc. There may be fine hæmorrhages in the macular region, which sometimes presents also the stellate arrangement of sclerosed spots usually found in nephritic retinitis, but which is here, as a rule, incomplete. The appearances spread irregularly upon the retina, usually following the vessels. As the inflammation declines, the redness and swelling of the disc disappear, and it becomes grayish in color, approaching white. The arteries contract to whitish filaments, venous tortuosity persisting for a considerable period.

The usual result is complete or partial atrophy. Vision depends more upon the condition of the circulation than the appearance of the nerve tissue, and may remain surprisingly good for a considerable time, but is eventually seriously affected if not lost. Reduction of function acts first on the color sense, then on central perception, eccentric vision and the light sense, in the order named. The peripheral field is usually contracted, often seriously.

As a rule, the disease attacks both eyes, though one may be later than the other.

RETROBULBAR NEURITIS may occur with serious loss of vision, but presenting only some hyperæmia of the retinal vessels with circumscribed haziness in the region of the disc, the latter being blurred in its outline. A valuable symptom is that of pain experienced by the patient when the eyeball is pressed directly backward, although this is sometimes but slightly noticeable.

The disease may be partial with corresponding visual defect, and scotoma, either positive or negative or for color only, may be present.

ATROPHY OF THE OPTIC NERVE may result from pressure without inflammation. It also sometimes occurs in children from inherited syphilis, the disc being first reddened and its edges blurred, later passing over into progressive atrophy. Vision is usually somewhat affected at the beginning, sometimes seriously, becoming further reduced as the disease progresses.

Clinical History.—Paleness of the disc, beginning at the temporal side and extending until the whole papilla is of a faint bluish or greenish white, the absence of the normal rosy color resulting from atrophy of the capillary circulation. There is disappearance of the fine vessels and the larger trunks become much reduced in size, the arteries being first affected. Later atrophic excavation occurs, the surface of the disc sinking somewhat, until in some cases the lamina cribrosa may appear.

Vision is lost slowly and progressively. There is contraction of the visual field, which is usually irregular and sometimes in sectors. The early loss of color perception is a useful diagnostic point in doubtful cases.

AMAUROSIS occurs in infants and children as a consequence of hereditary syphilis.

HEMIANOPSIA may result from brain lesion, the variety depending upon the part affected.

The prognosis in affections of the optic nerve is generally grave.

Treatment.—A proper hygienic regimen should be enforced. Use of the eyes for all near work should be prohibited, and they should be protected from the effects of bright light by suitable glasses. The former method of confining the patient in a dark room is not now regarded with favor, and it is better practice to encourage open air exercise and other measures calculated to benefit the general health.

Diseases of the retina and optic nerve present few symptoms upon which to base a prescription, and the general conditions must in every case be utilized to the fullest extent to insure accuracy in the selection of the drug. In cases resulting from syphilis the ocular affection is very frequently due to intracranial lesions, and headache and other cerebral symptoms often occur, which, together with the mental condition and the aggravations and ameliorations constitute the best guide to the correct remedy.

Agaricus.—This drug is well worthy of a trial in cases of atrophy of the optic nerve. It was first used by Dr. Wm. E. Rounds, in the clinics of the New York Ophthalmic Hospital, and some remarkable results were obtained by giving it for considerable periods in doses of five drops of the tincture twice or three times a day.

Asafœt.—Severe, boring pains over the eyebrows. Pressure in the eyes. Burning in the eyes. Pressive pains in the forehead from within outward. Aggravation at night. Relief from pressure.

Aurum.—Pain and soreness in the bones of the head and around the eye, aggravated by pressure. Constitutional symptoms afford the best indications for the drug.

Belladonna.—May be useful in either retinitis or optic neuritis. The inflammation is usually of a high grade. The optic disc is more or less swollen and blurred in its outlines. Œdema of the retina may be present, as shown by a faint grayish haze, particularly in the region of the disc and macula. The retinal vessels are enlarged and tortuous. Photophobia. Throbbing, jerking headache. Aggravations: noise, motion, jar and contact. Relieved by pressure.

Bryonia.—Particularly adapted to serous forms of disease. Œdema of the retina. Vertigo on rising. Sharp or pressive pain, beginning over the eye, later extending to the occiput. Soreness when moving the eyeballs in the orbits. Headache in the morning when first beginning to move. Pain in the eyeball, especially violent when moving the ball. Aggravation from motion, on rising or stooping, from moving the eyes. Amelioration from lying quietly with the eyes closed.

Duboisia.—In a proving of this drug, made by the writer in 1880, a complete picture of retinitis was developed, with swelling, redness, and blurring of the edges of the optic disc and engorgement and tortuosity of the retinal vessels. A symptom which has since proved to be characteristic was a sharp pain above the eye, between the eyeball and the rim of the orbit.

Kali Iod.—Very useful in retinitis or neuritis from syphilis. Especially indicated where the choroid or vitreous is involved. General symptoms afford the best guide in its selection.

Mercurius should be useful in diseases of the retina and optic nerve, particularly when the condition present is *aggravated by the glare of fire*. Pains in or around the eye. Symptoms aggravated at night.

Nux. Vom.—We have seen cases of optic neuritis due to cerebral lesions, much benefited by this drug, when the characteristic headache was present, with morning aggravation. It is also an excellent remedy in atrophy of the optic nerve.

Pulsatilla—Pressive pain in the forehead above the orbits. Headache with aching pain in the eyes. Throbbing, pressive headache. Aggravation in the evening and when raising the eyes. Amelioration in the open air, in a cool place and when lying upon the back. The writer has cured a severe case of syphilitic retinitis of long standing with this remedy, the indications being the pains in the head and the relief in the open air.

CHAPTER XXIX.

LIDS, LACHRYMAL APPARATUS, ORBIT AND MOTOR NERVES.

LIDS.—The lids may be the seat of chancre, of secondary eruptions and ulcerations, and gummata. Chancre on the lids occurs from kissing or other impure contact, and is always accompanied by marked swelling and induration. When fully developed it presents the usual appearance, and swelling of the pre-auricular and submaxillary glands is present. Secondary manifestations may appear as papules, pustules or ulcerations, the latter may extend from adjacent parts or may attack the lid primarily, appearing at the margin and rapidly affecting the whole thickness of the lid, the resultant scar being the characteristic notch.

If the ulceration originates on the integument it may quickly perforate the lid and destroy the bridge of tissue separating it from the free border. It commonly begins as an irregular, nodular, somewhat sensitive elevation, which soon breaks down into a foul sore, with ragged edges, indurated base, deep, uneven excavation, and discolored, disagreeable secretion. The surrounding tissue will be more or less swollen and infiltrated, and red or livid in hue. In bad cases one or both lids may be entirely destroyed. The ulceration may be the sole manifestation occurring at the time, but the contrary is usually the case.

GUMMY INFILTRATION of the lids may occur as a blepharitis, the free border being the site of small nodular growths, which later undergo purulent degeneration, the ciliary margin becoming ulcerated and inflamed and the lashes falling out.

The disease is slow and very obstinate, remaining confined to the margin, or including, by extension, the entire lid, in the latter case constituting the rare affection known as gummy tarsitis, or the tarsitis may be the initial lesion, the free border being attacked secondarily.

TARSITIS is of slow development, affects one or both lids of the same side, and is a gradual induration and thickening of the tarsus, progressing steadily until sometimes an enormous degree of swelling obtains, the skin being tense and dark red from venous stasis, and the conjunctival lining hypertrophied.

The pain is trifling except when abscesses result from foci of purulent degeneration in the mass. After persisting for a considerable period the swelling gradually subsides, leaving the tarsus of normal size or slightly shrunken.

The essential characteristics are the great hardening and thickening of the tarsus. The disease frequently lasts for many months but may terminate in perfect recovery.

Treatment should be same as that applied to like conditions occurring elsewhere.

LACHRYMAL APPARATUS. — DACRYOCYSTITIS

may be caused by the extension of specific disease of the nasal passages to the nasal duct or may be a resulting complication of syphilitic disease of the lachrymal bone. It may appear in either the acquired or hereditary form, the latter being the usual cause in cases occurring in young children.

When it follows nasal disease the mucous membrane of the nasal duct becomes swollen, possibly granular, with excess of secretion, consisting of mucus or muco-pus. In other cases syphilitic ulcerations of the nose may invade the duct, causing firm stricture by cicatricial contraction. As a result of these conditions, the secretions collect in the lachrymal sac, distending it and forming a tumor below the eye at the inner canthus. For a time the secretions may be freely pressed out at the puncta with the finger, but as the disease progresses and the calibre of the lachrymal passages becomes reduced by increased swelling it is impossible to entirely empty the sac in this manner, and the retained discharge may become irritating and even offensive. The natural outlet for the tears being closed, the eye becomes suffused and the tears flow over the cheek whenever the lachrymal secretion is stimulated, as by cold winds, etc. Later this condition becomes almost constant, interfering with vision and causing irritation and hypertrophy of the conjunctival lining of the lower lid, and sometimes blepharitis.

Acute aggravations take the form of abscess of the lachrymal sac, with severe pain, intense swelling, redness and exquisite sensitiveness of the part. As soon as pus is formed it should be given free outlet through the natural passages by an incision through the punctum and canaliculus into the sac, otherwise the abscess will rupture externally and may leave a permanent fistula upon the cheek.

In syphilitic cases, periostitis of the nasal or lachrymal bones is a frequent complication, and a permanent fistula may result from caries, or the disease of the bone may be the primary lesion, the affection of the lachrymal passages occurring by extension. Suppuration of the sac may occasionally result from degeneration of a gumma in this situation.

Treatment.—If stricture be present, it may be treated by dilatation by graduated probes passed through the punctum and canaliculus, or by electrolysis, a small probe attached to the negative pole being placed in the stricture, and three to six cells being used, until the probe is freely movable. By repeating this procedure, increasing the size of the probe at each sitting until a No. 5 can be easily passed, the case will soon be under control, after which astringent solutions may be injected to restore the mucous membrane to its normal condition. Where the above means fail, it may be necessary to incise the stricture after Stilling's method, as laid down in the text-books.

The principal remediesare Pulsatilla, Silicea and Stannum in the chronic form, and Hepar Sulph. will usually be called for in the acute aggravations.

PRE-LACHRYMAL ABSCESS, a disease which occupies substantially the same site, but which has no connection with the more deeply situated lachrymal sac, sometimes occurs in children as the result of hereditary syphilis.

DACRYO-ADENITIS OR INFLAMMATION OF THE LACHRYMAL GLAND, a very rare form of disease, may be a syphilitic complication. It is characterized by dull pain referred to the upper and outer portion of the orbital margin, with tenderness of the bone and the soft parts and swelling of the lids. On turning the upper lid the enlarged gland will appear as a tumor in the superior cul de sac.

The inflammation may disappear by resolution, by suppuration, or it may pass over into the chronic form. Sometimes the disease is chronic at the outset or there may be only simple induration. It may be bi-lateral.

Treatment does not differ from that of other glandular affections.

THE ORBIT.—PERIOSTITIS OF THE ORBIT

occurs principally in adults and belongs to the tertiary period of syphilis. It is also seen in children as a result of hereditary disease, though uncommon.

It is usually chronic, but may be acute and go on to suppuration. It may be marginal or occupy the deeper portions of the orbit; the deeper the situation the more serious the disease, especially in the acute form, which is particularly dangerous when it affects the roof. In the acute form, when marginal, there is usually a spot somewhere on the edge of the orbit, which is swollen and somewhat sensitive to pressure, and the pain is referred to this region. The pain is aggravated at night and may be severe; there is some chemosis, and swelling and redness of the lids; the motion of the eyeball toward the affected part is restricted, such effort causing a feeling of stiffness and pain.

If there is much swelling the eyeball may be displaced in the opposite direction. Diplopia is often present. Later an abscess may form, which should be opened as soon as fluctuation is detected, this treatment often resulting in speedy recovery.

When the disease attacks the deeper portions of the orbit, cellulitis may occur, with exophthalmus, general pain and tenderness on pressure, and more or less immobility of the ball. Here the diagnosis may be difficult.

The chronic form is usually slow and insidious, with the same symptoms in a lesser degree. Suppuration is, as a rule, slight, but may be considerable, and there is swelling and thickening of the periosteum; caries and sometimes necrosis may follow.

The disease may cause meningitis or abscess of the brain by extension, it may go on to resolution with entire recovery, or it may result in either exostosis or general thickening of the bones of the orbit, with consequent protrusion of the eyeball, paralysis and neuralgic affections from pressure.

Treatment.—Suppuration should be prevented if possible by the exhibition of the appropriate remedy, but when once fluctuation is detected the pus should be freely evacuated. If disease of the bone supervene a sufficient opening should be maintained to allow of thorough irrigation and disinfection of the parts, for which purpose solutions of Carbolic acid, 1 to 200, or Hydrarg. bi-chlor., 1 to 2000, will be found useful.

The drugs usually indicated are, in the order of their importance, Kali iod., Mercurius, Aurum, Asafœt. and Silicea.

MOTOR NERVES.—About one-half of the cases of ocular paralysis are believed to be due to some variety of syphilitic lesion. The affection may begin in the nuclei at the origin of the nerve supplying the part; the nerve trunk may be the subject of syphilitic infiltration or inflammation at some point in its course; it may be involved in specific inflammation of other parts, as in meningitis, or, finally, it may suffer from pressure as in gummata or exostoses. The resulting paralysis may be confined to a single muscle or may embrace the entire distribution of a nerve, as the lesion is situated in the trunk of the latter or in one or more of its branches. In some cases more than one nerve may be included in the destructive process.

Third Nerve—Motor Oculi.—If the lesion include the entire distribution of this nerve, the ciliary muscle, the sphincter iridis, the superior, inferior, and internal recti, the inferior oblique and the levator palpebra muscles will be paralyzed. As a consequence the eye will be turned outward and somewhat downward, from the unopposed action of the normal external rectus and superior oblique. Accommodation will be nil, the eye being adjusted for its far point; the pupil will be dilated and motionless; ptosis will be present, the upper lid hanging down over the cornea, rendering vision impossible except by manual interference, and a slight degree of exophthalmus may result from the relaxation of the paralyzed muscles; there will be crossed diplopia, the image of the affected eye being received at a point external to the macula lutea and projected in the opposite direction; or diplopia may be absent, the images being so far apart that only one can be appreciated.

If the lesion be limited to certain branches of the nerve its manifestations will vary accordingly.

Sixth Nerve.—This nerve supplies the external rectus muscle. If the paralysis be monocular, in attempting to look straight ahead the affected eyeball will turn inward, from the unopposed action of the normal internal rectus. On looking in the direction of the paralyzed muscle there will be a limitation of mobility dependent upon the degree of paralysis; the diplopia will be homonymous; the images will usually be on a level, and they will be farthest apart when looking in the direction of the paralyzed muscle, while the false image may disappear when looking to the opposite side.

Fourth Nerve.—This supplies the superior oblique muscle, which turns the eyeball downward and outward, and rotates the upper end of the vertical meridian inward.

Diplopia from paralysis of this muscle is greatest when looking downward, objects appearing double and irregular, one image is higher than the other and only one is vertical, the other being slanted obliquely.

In looking downward and inward the difference in height in the two images is greatest, but the obliquity of the false image is least, while in looking downward and outward the difference in height is lessened and the obliquity increased. The double images are homonymous and one appears nearer to the patient than the other. There is no diplopia above the horizontal median line.

In lesions of the third nerve the diplopia is most annoying for near objects, while in affections of the fourth and sixth nerves distant vision is the most troublesome.

As a result of the diplopia there may be nausea, vertigo and inability to correctly locate objects, which the patient tries to overcome by closing one eye or inclining the head. The difficulty may be palliated by using prisms pending treatment. Both eyes may be affected. The condition is obstinate and when of central origin the prognosis is grave.

Treatment should be directed toward the constitutional lesion.

CHAPTER XXX.

TERTIARY SYPHILIS.

This rarely shows itself until near the end of the second year; it has been known to appear as late as fifty-five years after the original chancre, the intervening condition being one of perfect health. This stage is characterized by infiltration of the tissues with a new cell growth, which increases at the expense of the infiltrated tissue, and degenerates rapidly on account of its low grade or want of organizing power, though it may be absorbed without apparent loss of continuity. When the skin or mucous membrane is involved it usually breaks down, forming deep ulcerations which tend to erode and destroy the surrounding tissue; these ulcers do not heal of themselves, and when cicatrization occurs deep scars and much loss of tissue often result. The same is true when it involves other portions of the body. These lesions are usually accompanied by cachexia, which is recognized by emaciation, loss of appetite and strength, mental depression, dry and tawny skin, dryness of the hair, sleeplessness, small rapid pulse, general anæmia, etc. Sometimes they respond kindly to hygienic and drug treatment, though in many cases the most perfect hygienic care and medication utterly fail; however, with the more modern understanding of the disease and its proper treatment during the early and secondary stages, tertiary conditions are now rare.

TERTIARY CUTANEOUS DISEASES.—Ecthyma may appear on any part of the body, but more frequently on the lower extremities; recovery is slow and successive evasions are liable to occur. It consists of an infiltration of the true skin, with a gummatous formation; after a few days a pustule appears on the solid elevation, breaking or drying into a dark brown or greenish crust which overlaps the original lesion, while beneath it the gummatous deposit breaks down forming an ulcer with sharp, abrupt edges, pultaceous floor and surrounded by a red areola of inflammation. On healing it leaves a depressed and deeply pigmented scar, which in time clears from the centre towards the circumference, leaving a pearly-white, lustrous spot.

Rupia occurs only when the system is profoundly affected by the syphilitic poison, the spots appearing isolated or in groups on any part of the body, and varying from one-third to an inch in diameter. They commence as pustules or vesicles which dry or rupture, forming a crust resting on an indurated base, and beneath it an ulcerating surface, discharging much pus. After a time the ulcer, by eating at its circumference, undermines the original crust which is raised by the constantly accumulating pus. This process is continued until layer after layer is formed, sometimes attaining an inch in thickness and resulting in a corrugated scab of a blackish or greenish-brown color; the ulcerating surface may finally heal underneath, or the crust may fall off, leaving a deep ulcer with abrupt edges and pultaceous base. When healed a deeply pigmented scar remains which finally becomes pearly-white from the centre to the circumference.

Pustules commence as small red spots soon becoming blisters which in a short time rupture or coalesce forming a thick greenish scab covering the whole of the affected surface and surrounded by a purplish-red areola. Beneath this crust ulceration goes on, extending beyond the circumference; it may fall off leaving a deep, ragged ulcerating surface that tends to extend superficially by serpiginous ulceration. On healing it leaves a deep-brown scar which in time whitens from the centre towards the circumference.

Ulceration of the cutaneous tissues in tertiary syphilis may be superficial or deep, the result of the breaking down and disintegration of the rapid cell-growth within the tissue.

The Superficial Ulceration usually originates as an ecthyma, rupia or pustule, gradually eating into the tissues beneath the crust which covers it. It may commence as a shiny red tubercule, one-quarter to three-quarters of an inch in diameter, which after a time breaks down and ulcerates. The ulcerations have abrupt adherent edges, pultaceous base, discharge a grumous pus and are usually covered with a greenish-brown scab. They are surrounded by an indurated copper-colored areola and may be stationary or serpiginous in character. They ulcerate at the circumference in curved lines, and on healing leave an irregular, deeply pigmented scar, which in time becomes white and glistening.

The deep variety of ulceration appears especially on the nose, ears, lips and the head of the penis, commencing as small tubercules that rapidly disintegrate; the ulceration eats deeply into the tissues beneath, destroying everything in its course, skin, connective tissue, muscle, cartilage and bone. These ulcerations are usually covered with a thick greenish-brown scab. The ulceration is sometimes intermittent in activity and leaves on healing a deeply pigmented scar which ultimately becomes white and glistening. Constitutional disturbances and pain are absent.

Gummata of the skin are sub-cutaneous infiltrations of the connective tissue by a small-celled granular gelatinous substance containing some fusiform cells and small blood vessels. These gummatous infiltrations are usually circumscribed, but may be diffuse, they are painless and at first are movable under the skin, but after a time become attached to the integument, a purplish point appearing upon the growth indicating inflammation. It then becomes sensitive, painful and ruptures, discharging a thick, bloody pus, etc., resulting in a specific ulcer with undermined edges, which may or may not heal. These gummata may be located on the head, neck or extremities.

Gummatous deposits also develop beneath the periosteum of the tibia, ulna, sternum, clavicle, skull, etc., differing from those under the skin only by being attached to the bone. They are sometimes followed by a slight necrosis of the osseous tissue and may burrow laterally instead of pointing and opening externally.

Treatment.—The general building up of the system by nutritious food, good hours, freedom from excessive mental and bodily excersise, outdoor employment, change of air, thermal baths, etc., are of the utmost importance. When ulcerations are present crusts and other exfoliated matter must be removed and the ulcer cleansed with a solution of Bichloride of Mercury (1–2000 to 20,000), or Hydrogen per-oxide, one part to three of water, or a one per cent. solution of Pyrozone and then dusted with Iodoform, Aristol, Dermatol, Calomel, Mercurius sol. 1x, Bismuth subnitrate, etc. Curetting and touching with Carbolic acid may be necessary.

Remedies.—Kali iod, Asafœtida, Aurum, Calcarea carb, Mezereum, Staphisagria, Sulphur, Thuja, Acid Nitric, etc.

CHAPTER XXXI.

LESIONS OF THE MUCOUS MEMBRANES IN TERTIARY SYPHILIS.

MUCOUS PATCHES may occur, and scaly patches are frequent.

DEEP ULCERATIONS are common, especially on the buccal mucous membrane, arch of the palate and the posterior and superior walls of the pharynx. They are surrounded by a dark-red collar, similar to the areola of the cutaneous lesions. The discharge from the ulcers is corrosive, irritating and scanty.

Gummatous ulceration of the mucous membrane is the most serious and rapidly destructive lesion of syphilis. It consists of an infiltration into the sub-mucous tissue of a gummatous material, either circumscribed or diffuse, and may be connected with or situated beneath the adjacent periosteum of the bony walls of the pharynx, the hard palate, vomer or bones of the face. The growth at first appears as a yellowish swelling, not sensitive to touch, soon icnreases in size, becoming oedematous, and red or purple in color. It ruptures and discharges a grumous substance, leaving a deep ulcer somewhat yellow in color, with red base and infiltrated edges. The ulcer degenerates and eats rapidly in the surrounding tissues, and may in one day destroy the hard and soft palate, the vomer, ethmoid, turbinated bones, etc., or it may extend upward and enter the cranial cavity, causing epilepsy, etc. The ulceration is, as a rule, unattended with pain unless there is some external irritation, as in the act of swallowing food and fluids, which are frequently regurgitated through the nose.

Treatment.—Cleanliness, disinfectants, antiseptics, dusting with Iodoform, together with the administration of Kali iod, Asafœtida, Mercurius, Aurum, Kali bich., Acid Nitric. Sanguinaria, etc.

CHAPTER XXXII.

LESIONS OF THE TONGUE, LARYNX AND LUNGS.

GUMMATA OF THE TONGUE may develop at any time during the secondary or tertiary stages of syphilis. These growths are located upon the upper surface and sides of the tongue, never on the under part. Gummatous infiltrations commencing deep in the muscular tissue, are painless, and, as they develop, the mucous membrane becomes elevated, stretched and slightly purple in color; they usually point at the centre and discharge, leaving a deep irregular but circumscribed ulcer. While much tissue may be destroyed, the ulcer eventually heals. It differs from epithelioma of the tongue in commencing deep in the muscular tissue and working outward, while epithelioma of the tongue commences on the surface and eats inward. The glands of the neck are not involved in gummatous ulceration of the tongue.

Treatment.—Gargles of Bi-chloride of Mercury, 1 to 5000, or the daily spraying of the ulcer with a solution of Nitrate of Silver, and finally dusting the surface with Iodoform will be required.

Remedies.—Kali iod., Mercurius, Acid Nitric., Silicea, Sulphur.

THE LARYNX is frequently involved in both secondary and tertiary syphilis; few escape lesions in this locality at some period of the disease.

Laryngeal Erythema may involve the whole or part of the larynx and is not attended with symptoms of any special character beyond a slight hoarseness.

Superficial Ulcers of the larynx occur late in the secondary stage; they are oval in form, surrounded by a deep red areola; their base is red, smooth, and covered with a grayish-yellow matter. They may be located on one or both sides of the larynx, causing hoarseness and other laryngeal symptoms; relapses are common. When the epiglottis is involved, deglutition becomes difficult. In neglected cases of syphilis the larynx above the vocal cords is especially liable to become involved and infiltrated with a growth, which contracts and greatly distorts the form of the larynx, giving rise to marked hoarseness and aphonia; sometimes these growths ulcerate.

Tertiary Laryngeal Symptoms may appear during the third year; they have been known to occur as late as forty years after the original invasion, appearing as gummatous ulcerations, vegetations, œdema and necrosis of the parts, finally resulting in stenosis, deformity and great impairment of the usefulness of the organ.

Deep Ulcers of the Larynx are usually single, but may be numerous; they are the result of gummatous infiltration and degeneration of the parts. The ulcers are deep, with sharp, adherent edges, and the floor is covered with a dirty, yellowish-white deposit, the tissue surrounding it being purple in color. The epiglottis rarely escapes and the cartilage of the larynx may be involved. If the epiglottis alone is diseased there will be no marked change in the voice, but it is usually somewhat impaired and there may be complete aphonia. Pain is generally absent, but the cough is troublesome, accompanied by profuse expectoration of pus, blood, broken-down tissue, etc. Respiration is greatly interfered with by œdema, growths and contraction of the cicatricial tissue. Excitement, exercise, etc., may bring on paroxysms of asthmatic, convulsive cough.

Prognosis.—Unless there is marked and progressive destruction of tissue the prognosis is good, although œdema or exhaustion may prove fatal. In all cases there will be permanent impairment of the larynx with consequent hoarseness.

Treatment.—The larynx should be kept clean by spraying it three or four times daily with a solution of Borax, Bicarb. of Soda (four or five grains to the ounce of warm water) or Dobell's solution; this affords much comfort to the patient. The ulceration should receive daily applications of a solution of Iodine, five to fifteen grains to the ounce of Glycerine, or a solution of Nitrate of Silver, five to thirty grains to an ounce of water, can be applied every few days. Rapidly supervening œdema will require tracheotomy. Moderate exercise, fresh air, good nourishment, massage, etc., are always advisable. Mercurius sol. or Mercurius corr. are indicated for the erythema and early ulcerations; Kali iod. for deep ulceration, gummata and œdema; Aurum when the bones and cartilage are affected, associated with mental depression; Nitric acid for sharp sticking pains in the larynx, offensive expectoration and hoarseness; Mezereum, Hepar sulphur and Kali bich. are frequently called for in special conditions and Sulphur in neglected cases with fibrinous indurations.

THE LUNGS may become involved either through acquired or hereditary syphilis.

White hepatization is an hereditary syphilitic pulmonary affection, found only in new born infants and commencing during intra-uterine life. A single lobe or the whole lung may be involved. The alveolar walls are thickened and infiltrated, the alveoli themselves being filled with large fatty and swollen epithelial cells. On section the lung is grayish-white in color and sinks in water. The infant lives but a few hours or days after birth.

Fibrinous Interstitial Pneumonia occurs in adults from acquired syphilis. It consists of an interstitial infiltration and induration of the interstitial tissue, which from its contraction may in time cause obliteration of the air cells and consequent deformity of the lung. On section the pulmonary tissue cuts like cartilage, yellow points are noticed upon its cut surface, the thickened walls of the bronchial tubes are dilated and distorted and the lung tissue does not crepitate.

Gummata of the Lungs may and usually do complicate specific fibrinous pneumonia. These infiltrations vary greatly in size, often becoming as large as an egg, are gray or grayish-red in color and are surrounded by consolidated lung tissue; they may become encapsulated and are white in color, or, more commonly, break down and open into the pleura or the nearest bronchus. There are no special signs or symptoms that distinguish this specific lesion of the lungs from tubercular or catarrhal phthisis, but the specific history, which should always be considered and treated accordingly.

CHAPTER XXXIII.

LESIONS OF THE ALIMENTARY TRACT.

STOMACH.—During the secondary stage erythema of the mucous membrane of the stomach sometimes occurs, causing indigestion, nausea and other functional disorders of a few days' duration.

Treatment.—Bland broths with Mercurius, Arsenicum or Nux vomica.

INTESTINES.—Gummatous growths may occur in the intestinal walls and break down, leaving round or oval ulcerations, which may open into the peritoneum or may heal, always leaving the characteristic specific scar. They are recognized by the history, cachexia and the diarrhœa which is difficult to control, the stools being frequently black and accompanied by pain, generally referred to the region of the gummatous ulceration; there is sometimes indigestion.

Treatment.—Diet: Kumyss, matzoon, broths, liquid peptonoids. Remedies: Kali iod., Kali bich., Mercurius corr., etc.

RECTUM.—Late in the tertiary stage of syphilis, broad, linear, gummatous infiltrations of the sub-mucous tissue of the rectum may occur, which on examination shows flat, livid, unulcerated and semi-elastic bands extending along the length of the rectum, frequently accompanied by vegetations, ulcers or mucous patches of the anus. As the infiltration and induration advances, stricture of the rectum is produced by the contraction of the newly formed tissue. Above the stricture the rectal mucous membrane is livid, excoriated and even ulcerated and attached to the muscular tissue by infiltrated growths and is less distensible than normal.

Clinical History.—The stools are at first small, frequently accompanied by mucus and blood; they finally become small, flat, ribbon-like and enveloped with mucus.

Treatment.—If recognized early the specific medication, if pushed, will cure the case; later, injections of thin flaxseed tea give much relief. If ulcers are present they will require cleansing with a Mercury bi-chloride, Pyrozone or Hydrogen-peroxide solution and dusting with Calomel, Iodoform or Aristol, or the three last can be used in the form of suppositories. When the stricture is excessive operation will be necessary.

Remedies.—Mercurius, Kali iod.

ANUS.—This may be the seat of erythema, papules, mucous patches, vegetations, ulcers, etc., requiring general or local treatment.

LIVER.—Diffuse Parenchymatous Hyperplasia is the most frequent lesion of hereditary syphilis. It consists of an infiltration of the parenchyma and vessels, the liver cells being compressed and distorted by its presence; it does not degenerate nor break down, but the liver becomes greatly enlarged and tense, hard and resistent, having the color of flint. In acquired syphilis the hyperplasia is circumscribed and results in a deep cicatrix which greatly distorts the liver and may divide it into two parts, the tissue between them being normal. In old syphilitics it may be in a state of amyloid or fatty degeneration.

Gummata.— May be single or scattered throughout the liver, varying from one-sixteenth to two inches in diameter. When located upon the surface of the liver they form nodules; when more deeply situated they cause contraction and puckering of the surface; the capsule of the liver is always thickened. The gummata undergo degeneration and are surrounded by dense, interlacing connective tissue which may extend through the liver.

Clinical History.—Percussion and palpation reveal a liver enlarged, cicatrized, irregular and nodular accompanied with pain, jaundice and specific cachexia; sometimes there is albuminuria, though the symptoms are not characteristic except when taken in conjunction with the syphilitic history.

Treatment.—Remedies: Mercurius in some of its forms, Kali iod., Hepar sulphur, etc.

THE SPLEEN may have connective tissue and gummatous deposits; there is no special clinical history.

Treatment.—Mercurius, Kali iod., Ceanothus.

KIDNEYS.—Simple Congestion.—In from eight to twelve weeks after the original chancre a slight congestion of the kidneys, a possible simple erythema of the uriniferous, tubules may occur. The urine becomes scanty and contains albumen, epithelial and granular casts. There is a general feeling of malaise, puffiness under the eyes or the œdema may be general; it disappears in a few days.

Treatment.—Mercurius corr. is usually indicated for this condition.

Syphilitic Nephritis.—In the later stages of syphilis gummata, interstitial hyperplasia and amyloid degeneration often develop without special symptoms except the presence of albumen and casts in the urine. If a specific history is given, good results may be expected from anti-syphilitic treatment, milk, mixed diet, good hours and hygiene.

CHAPTER XXXIV.

LESIONS OF THE BONES, CARTILAGES, MUSCLES AND TENDONS.

BONES AND CARTILAGES are often involved in both the secondary and tertiary stages of syphilis. Gummatous infiltrations may be circumscribed or diffuse. They are always accompanied by great sensitiveness and pain, especially at night. These specific nodes may be re-absorbed or break down with necrosis and loss of bony tissue. The flat and long bones lying near the surface are the most frequently involved. There is also a condition of dry necrosis without appreciable symptoms.

Treatment.—Kali iod, Mercurius, Aurum, Silicea, Mezereum, Asafœtida, Sulphur, etc.

MUSCLES AND TENDONS.—**Specific rheumatism** is not infrequent. It is usually mono-articular and characterized by the tender, painful points around the joints, with nocturnal aggravation.

Gummatous Infiltration of the fingers and toes are frequent, especially in the hereditary form of the disease.

The phalanges gradually and insidiously enlarge with or without much pain, the skin becoming purplish-red from infiltration, sometimes from hydro-arthrosis. If not treated in time it may become a pyriform tumor, which breaks down and discharges, leaving sinuses, or the bone sometimes shortens and becomes greatly atrophied.

Treatment.—The rheumatic condition can be relieved by some stimulating liniment or the application of Capsicum vaseline rubbed well into the parts, and internally Kali iod., or Mercurius in its various forms. The infiltrations may require in addition Nitro-muriatic acid, Hepar sulphur, Hekla lava, Phytolacca, etc.

CHAPTER XXXV.

NERVOUS SYSTEM.

Numerous disturbances of the nervous system occur as the result of the varied pathological changes which take place in and around the nerve centres and trunks from specific growths, ostitis, periostitis, etc. Gummata of various sizes develop and press on the nerve mass, the brain, meninges, pia mater, dura mater and arachnoid, which may be involved individually or collectively, producing numerous manifestations. Gummatous deposits may be distributed through the brain substance, varying from the smallest appreciable point to one or two inches in diameter, when numerous they are usually small and are associated with changes in the meninges. The larger ones are most frequently located in the walls of the ventricles, in the optic thalami, the corpora striata or in the white substance of the spinal cord. They are of yellowish-white color, cheesy in the centre, firm and hard externally, and are frequently surrounded by inflamed and softened brain tissue. The coats of the vessels of the brain and nervous centres may also become inflamed and infiltrated, often symmetrically, causing obstruction and leading to the red or white softening which occurs in non-specific thrombosis. These and many other changes give rise to many nervous symptoms ranging from cephalalgia to the more serious brain lesions.

CEPHALALGIA is one of the early symptoms of syphilis, and varies greatly in duration and intensity. It is often associated with disturbances of the special senses and digestive apparatus. The pain may be general or confined to the parietal, temporal or occipital region. It may be continuous or transitory and is always aggravated at night; some describe it as being of the most agonizing character, making the approach of night much to be dreaded. When the pain is localized the affected region is sometimes sensitive to the touch. These cases are usually amenable to some form of Mercury, Spigelia, Antipyrine or Phenacetine. If not relieved the special senses become affected, followed by loss of sleep, vertigo, impaired memory, apathy, melancholia, and finally they become bedridden and apparently afflicted with a hopeless cerebral lesion. With a specific history, however, there is yet hope, as many have recovered their mental faculties and strength to again become useful members of society by the aid of good hygiene, Mercurius, and appreciable doses of Kali iod.

HEMIPLEGIA is characterized by its incompleteness. The attacks are slight and usually occur without loss of consciousness, coming and going at short intervals, and often preceded by localized cephalalgia and tenderness over the affected cerebral region, neuralgic pains, numbness of the affected parts and lassitude. The hemiplegia may occur during the night or day; motor-function is not entirely lost, one arm or one leg may be involved, or only a certain group of muscles, or the arm and leg of one side and the facial muscles of the other. Hemiplegia occurring before the fiftieth year is very likely to be of specific origin.

The hemiplegia of syphilis is frequently accompanied by paralysis of one or more of the motor-oculi nerves, which is pathognomonic of syphilis. There are cases in which motor-oculi paralysis may be the only evidence of intra-cranial disease; the reason of the frequency of this condition is due to these nerves lying in contact with the meninges and the floor of the skull for a long distance before entering the orbit where specific deposits frequently occur. If it is syphilitic, the prognosis is good compared to a similar condition resulting from other causes.

Treatment.—General care as adapted to the requirements of each case.

Remedies.—Mercurius or Kali iod.

FACIAL PARALYSIS may occur early or late in syphilis, and is sometimes preceded by formication, numbness, etc. In late syphilis it may indicate the approach of hemiplegia.

APHASIA, which is a common manifestation in late syphilis, may be transitory or continuous and has no special symptom to mark it, except the general history, which, when present, greatly improves the prognosis. When the victim speaks two languages he may be unable to converse in one, but can speak the other, or when unable to speak at all can write his wishes and desires.

Treatment.—Mercurius and Kali iod.

CHOREA.—Choreiform movements may be present either before or after a paralytic seizure, and may be of long or short duration.

EPILEPSY is usually preceded by headache, etc. The seizure may be heralded by prodomal symptoms. In the *grand mal* of specific epilepsy the shrill cry of true epilepsy is absent; unconsciousness is never complete; there may be frothing at the mouth. The seizures occur at intervals of hours, days or weeks, and lead in time to dementia. Syphilitic epilepsy occurs usually in adults who have a specific history and have not had epileptic fits before their twenty-fifth year. In specific epilepsy the seizure usually lasts half an hour or more, while true epilepsy usually commences in childhood, and the convulsive seizure rarely lasts over five minutes. The convulsion commences unilaterally in a finger or toe, thence extending over the body. The *petit mal* is a mild form in which only one set of muscles is involved, with perhaps momentary loss of memory, confusion of thought and incoherent speech.

PARAPLEGIA occurs without loss of consciousness; it may have been preceded by other specific nervous conditions and may be partial, complete, sudden or slow in development. Fifty per cent. of all cases of paraplegia occurring under forty years of age are of specific origin. It frequently occurs without sensory disturbance, one side of the body alone may be involved; the paralyzed muscles are subject to convulsive seizures and to localized hyperæsthesia and anæsthesia.

Treatment.—Mercurius, Kali iod., etc.

INSANITY.—Syphilis undoubtedly causes various forms of mental aberration, hence it is well to always look for the specific land marks and if evidence can be found of syphilis to give the patient the benefit of the doubt, and treat him accordingly.

COMA resulting from syphilitic lesions may be preceded by cephalalgia, anæsthesia, hyperæsthesia, paraplegia, hemiplegia, loss of memory, etc. It may appear suddenly during the night, when the patient will be found the following morning apparently asleep, but can be aroused to take food and drink, listless, yet able to answer questions and recognize friends; the pulse and respiration are slow, the pupils contracted, the eyeballs sunken and the eyes directed outward, with dry tongue, involuntary stools, and sub-normal temperature. These symptoms, together with the age of the patient, will be of great diagnostic importance.

Treatment.—Mercurius, Kali iod., Stramonium, etc.

CHAPTER XXXVI.

MARRIAGE AND PREGNANCY OF SYPHILITICS.

Marriage.—The male should not entertain the idea of contracting marriage until three years after the primary lesion and provided no specific symptoms have appeared during the third year. In the female, in whom the disease is less marked, the taint remains longer, and five years should intervene between the chancre and marriage, to be reasonably certain that it may result, if pregnancy occurs, in the birth of a healthy child. Some marry earlier without serious subsequent results. When properly treated there is no reason why all should not at some time marry, but while primary or secondary manifestations are present no one with any sense of right or justice should entertain for one moment the thought of marriage.

Syphilis in Pregnancy.—A woman suffering from the early manifestations of syphilis will surely abort at about the third month if the disease is not treated. Each succeeding pregnancy may go on a little later, until finally an apparently healthy child is born; but after a short time it may become shriveled, old mannish, without apparent cause, and finally dies. The miscarriage in the syphilitic mother is usually due to gummatous deposits, general or circumscribed, in the placenta. If the mother is placed under the proper anti-syphilitic treatment, and this is continued during pregnancy, a healthy child may always be expected, except during the first pregnancy, when abortion almost always results, even if the proper treatment is instituted.

The treatment must be continued through a number of successive pregnancies, because if neglected it will result in syphilitic offspring. Mothers of syphilitic children are usually the victims of syphilis, but not necessarily so. A syphilitic father may procreate a syphilitic child without contaminating the mother; a syphilitic mother with a non-syphilitic father may produce a syphilitic child, but under proper treatment healthy children can be and are born even if both parents are syphilitic. Cases are on record where healthy children have been born to syphilitic parents who have received no specific treatment; the mother should, however, always be treated during pregnancy, when a specific history is known and there is reason to believe that the disease has not been entirely eradicated. While it is rare for a parent with tertiary symptoms to produce a syphilitic child, cases have been recorded where syphilitic children have been born years after the original lesion.

Treatment.—Mercurius, Kali iod. and Kali muriaticum.

CHAPTER XXXVII.

HEREDITARY SYPHILIS.

Hereditary Syphilis.—Lesions in this form are discussed under separate heads, but some conditions presented in early hereditary syphilis require special consideration. When syphilis begins in utero, a miscarriage usually occurs and the child dies at birth or within a short period afterwards. One of the early evidences is coryza or snuffles with acrid discharge from the nose, mucous patches in the mouth, nose and larynx, causing the peculiar cry, which is harsh and irritating. Vegetations may appear at the various openings of the body. A roseola or papular rash is often noticed around and upon the buttocks, the skin is wrinkled, dry and lustreless, of a sallow or earthy color and drawn over the bony prominences, giving a prematurely aged look to the child, the hair is dry and scanty; in fact, the general appearance is that of marasmus with general syphilitic conditions. These children rarely survive the third month, but some live on to die later of syphilitic gummata or other diseases, but if they grow up they are stunted. Dentition is delayed, the permanent teeth presenting certain peculiarities that are pathognomonic and are known as Hutchinson's teeth; the upper central incisors are dwarfed, too short, too narrow, and if a single central cleft in their free edge is present the diagnosis is almost certain. When the dwarfing is absent, or if the peculiar dwarfing is present without cleft, there can be little doubt in the diagnosis. The nose, eyes, bones, joints and larynx are specially liable to show late hereditary symptoms. Hereditary syphilis, if present, almost always appears in some form or other before the sixth month.

Treatment.—The child must be nursed by the mother if her health is good, as Collie's law excludes all danger to her. If not, the Walker-Gordon laboratory prepared milk, made to agree with the child can be recommended, or the following can be given:

              Cream, ... ℥iss.
              Milk, ... ℥i.
              Water, ... ℥v.

To this add two teaspoonfuls of sugar of milk. Bottle in proper feedings. Heat to 167° F., cork tightly with absorbent cotton and place in refrigerator until wanted for use, then warm and add a half teaspoonful of lime water to each feeding. Malted milk, Carnrick's, Nestle's or Mellin's food, or condensed milk (not canned), diluted one to ten or seven, as required by the age of the child, can be used.

Remedies.—Mercurius sol. Hahn. is usually indicated, but if the stomach is in a specially depraved condition it is better to use mercurial inunctions.

CHAPTER XXXVIII.

TREATMENT OF SYPHILIS.

General Consideration.—Excesses of all kinds, physical or mental, must be interdicted; out-door employment and recreation are to be recommended, as well as short vacations in the country; the diet should be regulated to give the greatest amount of nourishment and the least work to the digestive apparatus, which is frequently somewhat impaired, hence it must be simple and non-irritating in character with meals at regular hours.

If lesions of the mouth or throat exist, very hot or very cold food should not be eaten, and if mercurials are being exhibited in appreciable doses, acids must be avoided. Alcohol may be allowed in moderation only; brandy and champagnes should always be prohibited, but burgundy, claret and other light wines, and ale, beer and porter may be taken in moderation with the meals. In every case the use of tobacco must be prohibited. If smoking and chewing are not discontinued, lesions will appear upon the mucous membrane of the mouth and throat, causing much pain and annoyance. Sleep should be regulated. The organs of the body must receive due attention and functional or organic diseases be properly treated. Cod liver oil in its various forms, panopeptones, peptonoids, somatose, etc., will be of great benefit in building up the constitution. The whole body must receive frequent and careful physical examinations. Proper clothing should be worn, not too warm causing fatigue or too light allowing chilling of the surface, etc. Flannels should be worn at all times. During treatment bathing must receive proper consideration, one or two Turkish baths weekly and sulphur or alkaline baths are of great benefit. Cold plunges in the morning, recommended and taken by so many, are frequently productive of shock to the system and weaken the body instead of strengthening it. The Hot Springs of Arkansas and other home and foreign springs of renown are frequently recommended, but the good results are due more to the compulsory regulation of habits, together with simple, wholesome food, than to the springs themselves; yet it is a well-known fact that those sojourning there can and do take much larger doses of the mercurials and iodides than they are able to at home; hence the apparent excellent results from visits to these springs. In all things moderation must be the rule; if restrictions are too rigid, the patient feels uneasy and discouragement often follows. Cases must remain under observation for at least three years; many are cured in less time, but scrofulous, gouty and other conditions frequently complicate and prolong the treatment. At one time, when many objected to mercurial treatment, excision of the chancre was practiced but without modifying in any way the general symptoms of the disease. Of remedies many have had their rise and fall, but only two, Mercury and Iodide of Potash, have stood the test of time and science; Mercury, alone or in combination, is indicated in most all of the secondary and many of the tertiary symptoms and under certain conditions in the primary stage, when the functions of the parts are interfered with or when fever, phagedæna, etc., seem to require it.

From the pathogenesis and symptomatology of this remedy we may expect and do receive the best of results, unless it has been unscientifically administered. Much of the patient's future and his immediate health will depend on the proper adjustment of the dose, and the selection of the appropriate preparation to the period and conditions presented. It is universally used, but the dose and mode of administration vary greatly. Hahnemann says Mercury is the specific remedy for syphilis. Yeldham advises

Merc. sol. 1x or 2x in five grain doses; also the Proto-iod. or Bin-iod. in the second and third decimal trituration. Jahr recommends Merc. sol. Hahn., Merc. præcip. rub. or Cinnabaris in one-half grain doses of the second trituration. Baehr prefers the Mercurius in the third decimal trituration. Jousset, the Merc. corr. Keyes uses Merc. proto-iod. in doses he calls tonic. Others believe in inunction of Mercurial ointment, and hypodermics of the bi-chlorides are also advised. No preparation of Mercury must be prescribed upon the stage or time that has elapsed since the chancre, and the same may be said of Kali iod., Aurum, Graphites, etc., for the tertiary symptoms are not always the late symptoms and the secondary are not always the early ones, but those who have been conscientiously and carefully treated with a mercurial preparation are rarely affected with tertiary symptoms.

Some of the special accepted modes of administration of Mercury are deserving of particular mention.

Keyes' Continuous Tonic Treatment has received much attention and has many followers. He advises the administration of granules containing 1-6 of a grain of the Proto-iodide of Mercury as follows: One after each meal for three days; on the fourth day add one granule to the noon dose; continue this for three days; then add one to the night dose; continue this for three days, finally increasing the morning dose and continue for three days; continue in this manner, being careful as to food, drink and exposure, until intestinal irritation, diarrhœa and colicky pains are produced, or until the gums show evidence of commencing mercurialization. When these symptoms occur they indicate that the dose last taken is the full dose which may be continued with Opium and unstimulating diet until the secondary symptoms yield. One-half of this dose is the tonic dose, which must be continued unceasingly month after month. Should any symptoms of syphilis appear the full dose may be given until they yield.

Inunction Treatment is indicated when the Proto-iodide or some other form of Mercury has been administered for some time and the secondary symptoms do not disappear. During this treatment the patient must be constantly watched; if he looks, feels and sleeps well, the medication is considered to be successful and should be continued. As a rule 20 to 45 grains of Mercurial ointment may be used daily, but in the robust and healthy one drachm is often necessary. In all cases at the beginning the patient must be examined daily to see that no unpleasant effects are produced, necessitating a reduction of dose or its discontinuance. The inunction should always be given by a professional masseur, though the patients may learn to do it themselves. A 20 per cent. Oleate of Mercury is sometimes substituted and used in the same quantity. Inunction can be administered night or morning, as best adapted to the circumstances of the patient. The region where inunction is to be given should first be washed with soap and warm water, then with a two per cent. solution of Carbolic acid (which should also be used after the weekly general bath); the hairy parts, as a rule, are not anointed, but if it becomes necessary to apply Mercury to these parts the hair should be removed before giving the inunction. When local medication is required and shaving of the parts is objectionable, the Ungt. hydrarg. ammoniatum may be substituted. In giving unctions gloves are not required by the operator, but a little sweet oil, simple cerate or soap, applied to the hands before beginning, and washed off immediately afterwards, is the only precaution necessary to prevent disease or salivation, provided always that the hands are in a healthy condition. The amount of ointment to be used should be divided into several parts and firmly and evenly rubbed into the selected region, combining friction and massage; the usual time required for each inunction is about twenty minutes, the skin looking on its completion as though it had been pot-leaded. When the inunction is completed suitable night clothes should be put on (to protect the bed linen), and the patients should retire and roll themselves in blankets to induce a gentle perspiration which is facilitated by taking a generous drink of hot milk or beef tea. The body is usually completely anointed in six sittings as follows: The back and neck, chest and abdomen, the right arm, the left arm, left leg, right leg (avoiding the scrotum); on the seventh day a hot bath should be taken and the inunction omitted. The number of inunctions varies according to the requirements of the individual case.

Fumigation has its advocates; its sphere is for emergencies only and not for continuous treatment. Twenty to forty grains of Calomel are placed over the fusing lamp (Fig. 38), or a combination of 15 grains of Calomel and 20

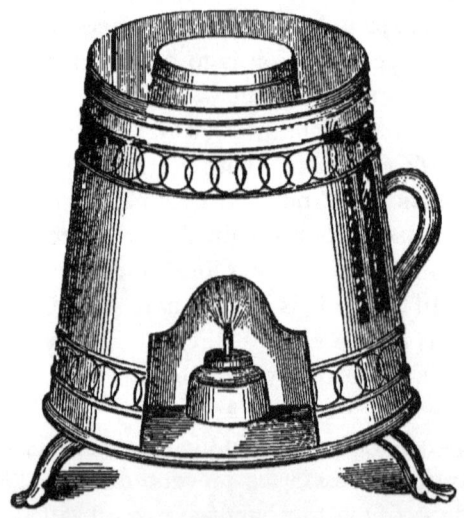

FIG. 38.

grains of Cinnabaris may be used; the quantity being diminished or increased as required. The selected mercurial is placed in the cup and about 4 ounces of water poured into the groove which surrounds it; the patient then sits on a chair, covered only with a blanket or mackintosh and the lamp is lighted. The heat and steam soon induce free perspiration, and the Mercury is deposited upon the surface of the body, the patient sometimes being allowed to breathe the fumes well mixed with air. When fumigation is complete the patient should retire and cool off slowly and remain in bed for some time. In cold weather attention to clothing after the treatment is necessary, and proper clothing must be worn when going out, to avoid taking cold, etc. These baths are best taken at bed time, but never immediately after a meal; if the patient is tired or debilitated after the bath the quantity of Mercury must be reduced or fumigation discontinued. Fumigation should not be administered daily; every second or third day usually gives the most satisfactory results, but it should never be continued more than one or two months.

Hypodermics of Mercury should not be used as routine treatment, though they are beneficial in many cases. While numerous compounds have been recommended, the bi-chloride undoubtedly acts best; 1-8 to 1-50 of a grain may be used diluted with 10 minims of distilled water. The usual anti- and aseptic precautions must be observed. After filling the syringe, place it in a five per cent. solution of Carbolic acid, and spray the skin in the region where the hypodermic is to be given with some of the same solution; the needle is then introduced into the subcutaneous tissue and the bi-chloride solution slowly injected, and on its removal it can be followed by slight massage of the part. The gluteal region should be selected, as its anatomical construction is considered best adapted for hypodermic injection. The hypodermic may be given every second day; pain and congestion may follow, but rapidly disappear.

To sum up, the mercurials most frequently required in the early period of the secondary stage are the Merc. sol. Hahn., Merc. vivus or Merc. proto-iod.; in the late secondary and tertiary syphilis, while the former are useful, Merc. bin-iod. and Merc. bichloride, Cinnabaris and Merc. dulcis will be more frequently indicated.

Iodide of Potash is the other remedy that has served well and cured many of the late manifestations of syphilis; all agree that the best results are obtained as a rule by the administration of the drug in appreciable doses, gradually increased. It is generally given in a saturated solution, each drop of the solution corresponding to 1 grain of the drug. It should be given in milk, after meals, the usual dose being 5 to 7 grains, although drachm doses every four hours have been administered successfully in cases of gummata of the brain. Sometimes in the intermediate stage between the secondary and tertiary, what is known as the mixed treatment is frequently administered with gratifying results; it consists of a combination of Mercury and Iodide of Potash. The following are good examples:

COMPRESSED TABLETS.

℞ Potassii Iod., ... gr. v.
Hydrarg. Chlor. Cor., ... gr. $\frac{1}{30}$.
Syr. Sarsapar. Comp., ... m. xxx.
M.

Ft. Tablet i.

Sig. One after each meal; increase dose according to requirements of case.

It can also be administered in liquid form:

LIQUID.

℞ Hydrarg. Bin-iod., ... gr. iii.
Potassii Iod., ... ʒiii v.
Syr. Sarsapar. Comp., ... ʒi.
Aqua, ... ad. ʒviii.
M.

Sig. A teaspoonful in a wineglassful of water after meals.

Others use the bin-iodide or the proto-iodide of Mercury in various potencies before meals and the appropriate quantity of the Iodide of Potash in milk or water after meals.

Hughes says "nothing will take the place of Iodide of Potash in the tertiary lesions of syphilis." Farrington says: "This remedy acts on the fibrinous and connective and finally the nerve tissues. The tendency of this drug is to produce infiltrations, so when thoroughly indicated there will be an œdematous or infiltrated condition of the part." This remedy is indicated in all of the late secondary and tertiary symptoms. When gummatous infiltrations take place it is our only safe anchor, whether they occur in the nervous system, the bones or elsewhere. In hereditary syphilis, the early coryza, etc., is greatly modified by this remedy.

Other remedies will be required as inter-currents for special conditions and complications, when the mercuries given for the early lesions or the Kali iodide in the later manifestations do not give satisfactory results.

CHAPTER XXXIX.

SPECIAL THERAPY FOR SYPHILIS.

Acid Fluoric.—Acts especially upon the bones and skin; caries of the bones, pains worse at night, of a burning and intermittent character; tubercules on the forehead and face; ulcerating squamous eruptions on the body; mucous tubercules, tertiary affections of the tongue; all discharges thin, acrid and excoriating.

Acid. Nitric.—Phagedænic ulceration on the tibia, etc.; ulcers with irregular edges, exuberant vegetation, bleed easily; copper-colored blotches on the skin; secondary syphilides, especially on the face; suppurating pustules on the face with broad red areola or covered with crusts; squamous eruptions like psoriasis; cracks and fissures around the commissures of the lips; fetid odor of the breath; mucous patches covered with well-marked white deposit; ulceration of the nostrils and throat with discharge;

ulcers and gummata of the mouth, uvula, pharynx and fauces; soreness of the tongue and its edges; ulceration of the rectum, with constipation.

Arsenicum.—Syphilitic cachexia; emaciation; debility, restlessness, anguish, excessive sensitiveness, general thinning of the hair, skin livid, with scaly eruption; tuberculous syphilides; malignant ulcerations; corrosive discharge with tendency to gangrenous destruction; fetid, exhausting, bloody diarrhœa with constant urging; evidence of serious intestinal disease.

Arsenicum Iod.—Syphilitic consumption.

Asafœtida.—Tertiary syphilitic lesions of the long bones; gummatous deposits; jerking drawing pains in the limbs, worse at night, ulceration of the skin with a thin, fetid, ichorous discharge; sensitive to touch.

Aurum.—Cachexia, depression with great mental weakness, despair and prostration; periostitis of the cranial and long bones; caries of the bones of the mouth and nose; soreness in the nose with swelling and loss of smell; putrid discharge from the nose; ulcers on the tongue; alopecia, pain in the bones worse at night; syphilitic orchitis.

Carbo Animalis.—Emaciation; periostitis; red, copper-colored blotches on the skin, especially on the face; tubercules of the skin; gummata; glands in various parts of the body enlarged and indurated; venous circulation sluggish, hands and feet blue and cold; gangrene.

Carbo Vegetabilis.—Specific cachexia, great debility and emaciation; copper-colored spots on the skin; tertiary syphilides; specific ulcerations of the skin, with thin, acrid and offensive discharge; gangrene, cold sweat, cold breath, collapse; ulcerations having cadaverous odor; lymphatic glands swollen, digestive organs impaired; skin of a yellow hue with shooting pains through the liver and spleen.

Cinnabaris.—Syphilitic catarrh, pressure at the root of the nose, feeling as though something was pressing on the nose; throat swollen, tonsils enlarged, red and congested;

chronic mucous patches on the mucous membrane of the mouth; small ulcers on the roof of the mouth and tip of the tongue; dryness of the throat and nose worse at night and on awakening; secondary syphilides of the mucous membrane.

Corallium Rub.— Coral-red spots on various parts of the body, especially on the palms of the hands, finally changing to a copper color; specific erosions exuding a thin badly smelling ichor.

Graphites.— Indolent ulcerations; specific psoriasis; chronic skin diseases; glandular swelling.

Hepar Sulphur.—Great nervous weakness, alopecia, painful swelling of the scalp; pains in the bones of the head, worse at night and from pressure, with red and inflamed eyes; tonsils swollen and hard with enlargement of glands of the neck; caries of the bones, especially of the face, with a discharge smelling like decayed cheese.

Iodum.—Syphilitic cachexia; pustular eruptions on the skin and secondary lesions of the mucous membrane.

Kali Bich.—Ulcers of the fauces and mouth that tend to perforate, surrounded by a copper-colored zone; deep ulceration of the tongue; scaly patches on the tongue; discharge of hard, green mucus from the throat, coughed up with difficulty from the posterior nares in the morning; ozœna and caries of the bones of the nose; ulcers spread superficially and not deeply; syphilitic laryngitis with dry, hoarse, barking cough; nodes on the cranium with deep pain in the osseous tissue; pustular and other tertiary eruptions with deep ulceration.

Kali Iod. is indicated in all the tertiary lesions of the skin, gummatous infiltration of the internal organs, and frequently in some of the secondary conditions found in hereditary syphilis. In scrofulous and debilitated constitutions; violent headache, with hard lumps on the head; alopecia; roseola, papular and pustular eruptions on the face, scalp, chest and body, that on healing leave a cicatrix; tertiary syphilides; rupia; discolored ulcers; gummatous infiltration of the nervous tissue and the internal organs with their local and reflex symptoms; foul breath, sore throat; ulceration of the bones of the nose; ozœna with greenish-yellow and exhausting discharge; ulcers eating deeply into the tissues and leaving large scars; gummatous infiltration of the bones and periosteum, these infiltrations have no fluctuations, but have a deep doughy feeling, with throbbing, gnawing, burning, boring pains, which are worse at night; enlarged glands in the groin, neck, etc.; infiltrations of the soft tissues and bones; ulceration of bones.

Lachesis.—Gangrenous and phagedænic chancres; sore throat; ulceration of the mouth and throat; ulcers surrounded by a bluish areola with constant inclination to cough, with itching and painful deglutition and regurgitation through the nose; violent pain in the head; pains in bones worse at night; flat ulcers on the lower extremities with bluish areola; pimples, pustules and ulcers with offensive discharge, skin around them mottled, blue-red; swelling along the course of the veins; discharge from the ulcers ceasing and the parts become cold and œdematous, patient cold and stupid with failing strength, dark blisters appear around the ulcers; caries of the tibia.

Lycopodium.—Depression of the nervous system; tearing, burning pains worse at night; dark grayish-yellow ulcers on the throat, especially the right side, with cough and hoarseness from similar ulcers on the larynx; face sallow; copper-colored eruptions on the forehead; ulcers of the leg sluggish and refuse to heal.

Mercurius.—The action of this drug is far-reaching. There are no lesions of the secondary stage that do not call for the administration of Mercury in some form, and many in the tertiary stage are greatly benefited by it. It diminishes the relative number of red corpuscles in the blood of the healthy person and is indicated and especially efficacious in the chloro-anæmia of syphilis, as well as in syphilitic fever, whether of the intermittent or catarrhal form; alopecia; pains in the bones are worse at night; round copper-colored and red spots on the skin; vesicles; erythema; papules and scaly eruptions; small ulcerations become covered with a crust, secrete a fetid pus; periosteum swollen, indurated and the skin over it unhealthy, with pain in the bone, restlessness, etc. *Merc. sol.* is indicated in congenital syphilis; erythematous, papular and squamous syphilides, especially on the palms, the spots are red and scale off; erythematous congestion of the pharynx and mucous membrane; syphilitic fever; all pains worse at night. The *Bin-iod.* is indicated for the Hunterian chancre, and the *Proto-iod.* for secondary syphilides, sore throat, alopecia, headache, etc. *Merc. corr.* for destructive, serpiginous ulcerations with ragged edges, eating rapidly; iritis; secondary syphilides; sore mouth and throat, especially when the uvula is swollen, red and elongated, with burning and violent constriction of the throat on any attempt to swallow liquids or solids, which causes a spasm and regurgitation of food; pulse quick and irregular; syphilis of internal organs. *Acid Nitrate of Merc.* will be of great benefit for the sticking pains in the throat, etc., with other mercurial symptoms.

Mezereum.—Local nocturnal pains; nodes on the tibia, chronic sore throat with dark redness of fauces, worse every winter, with burning and dryness down the larynx, hoarseness and hawking of phlegm.

Phosphorus.—Specific plantar psoriasis of hands and feet; roseola and squamous lesions of the skin; exostosis of the long bones, pains worse at night.

Phytolacca.—Weakness and depression; nodes on the face; whole body, including feet and face, etc., covered with pale red spots about the size of a dime. Secondary syphilides; rupia; pains in the long bones, worse at night, glands swollen; sore throat, ulcers in the throat; mucous patches.

Stillingia.—Specific affections of the long bones, with

gummatous deposits; ostitis and periostitis, pains worse at night; syphilitic ulcerations of the skin covered with crusts; enlarged cervical glands; specific ozœna; ulceration of the mouth and throat; discharge from the nostrils, excoriating the nose and upper lip; tubercular eruptions of the skin.

Staphisagria.—Syphilides; round, oval, whitish, raised spots on the mucous membrane of the mouth; syphilitic gummatous ulcerations, caries of the bones with thin discharge.

Sulphur.—Copper-colored spots on the forehead; tertiary syphilides.

INDEX.

A.

Abortive Treatment of Gonorrhœa, ... 45
Abortion from Syphilis, . . 285
Abscess of the Pelvis of the
    Kidney, ... 134
    Treatment of, ... 134
Acne, Syphilitic, ... 233
Adenitis, Inguinal, . . 46, 212
    Treatment of, . . . 46, 215
Alopecia, Syphilitic, ... 236
    Treatment of, ... 236
Amaurosis, Syphilitic, . . . 260
Anus, Syphilis of, ... 278
Aphasia, Syphilitic, . . . 283
Aspermatism, ... 188
Atrophy of the Optic Nerve,
    Syphilitic, ... 259
Atrophy of the Testicle, . . 156
Azoospermism, ... 188

B.

Bacillus of Lustgarten. . . . 220
Balano-Posthitis, ... 17
    Etiology of, ... 17
    Clinical History of, . . 17
    Prognosis in, ... 18
    Treatment of, ... 18
    Special Therapy for, . 26–33
Banks' Filiform Bougie, . . 60
Bastard Gonorrhœa, ... 36
    Etiology of, ... 36
    Clinical History of, . . 36
    Treatment of, ... 37
    General Treatment of, . 36
    Special Therapy for, . 64–73
Bates' Urethral Hæmostat, . 55
Bigelow's Lithotrite, . . . 127
Bigelow's Evacuator, . . . 128
Bladder, Acute Inflammation of, ... 101

Etiology of, ... 101
Pathological Anatomy
    of, ... 102
Clinical History of, . . 102
Treatment of, ... 103
Special Therapy for, 140–154
Bladder, Chorea of, ... 111
    Treatment of, ... 111
    Special Therapy for, 140–154
Bladder, Chronic Inflammation of, ... 103
    Etiology of, ... 103
    Pathological Anatomy
    of, ... 103
    Clinical History of, . . 105
    Treatment of, ... 107
    Special Therapy for, 140–154
Bladder, Irritability, of, . . 109
    Etiology of, ... 109
    Clinical History of, . . 109
    Treatment of, ... 110
    Special Therapy for, 140–154
Bladder, Irritation of the
    Neck of, in Gonorrhœa,
                   40, 102
    Treatment of, ... 40
Bladder, Stone in, ... 115
    Etiology of, ... 116
    Clinical History of, . . 116
    Non-operative Treatment of, ... 120
    Operative Treatment of, 121
    Stone in, in Females, . . 130
    Treatment of, ... 131
Blood in Syphilitics, ... 228
Blunt-pointed Meatotomy
    Knife, ... 50
Bones, Syphilis of, ... 280
    Treatment of, . . . 280
Böttcher's Crystals, ... 91

Bottini's Thermo-galvanic
  Cautery, for Hypertro-
  phy of the Prostate, . 100
Bougies, Bulbous, ... 44
Bougies, Banks' Filiform, 60
Brandt's Massage for Incon-
  tinence of Urine, . . 112
Bubo, ... 46, 212
  Simple Inflammatory, . . 212
    Clinical History of, . . 212
    Abortive Treatment of, 215
    Treatment of, . . . 46, 215
  Syphilitic, ... 214, 224
  Virulent, ... 214
    Treatment of, ... 215
    Enucleation of, ... 216
    Surgical Treatment of, . 216
    Special Therapy for, 217, 218
Bulbous Bougies, ... 44
Bulbous Syphilides, ... 234

C.

Cachexia, Syphilitic, . . . 28
Calculi, Renal, ... 137
Calculus, Vesical, ... 115
Cancer of the Penis, ... 21
  Etiology of, ... 21
  Clinical History of, . . 21
  Treatment of, ... 21
  Special Therapy for, . 26–32
Cancer of the Testicle, . . 172
  Treatment of, ... 173
  Special Therapy for, 179-184
Caries Dry, of Bones, Syphi-
  litic, ... 280
Cartilage, Syphilis of, . . . 280
Castration, ... 174
Catheter, Double Current, . 107
Catheter, English, ... 98
  Grooved-Tunneled, . . . 57
  Mercier's, ... 98
  Soft Elastic, ... 98
  Silver, with long Curve, . 98
Cephalalgia, Syphilitic, . . 282
Chancre, ... 221
  Differential Diagnosis of, . 224

Diphtheroid, ... 223
Dubuc, ... 223
Erosions of, ... 223
Hunterian, ... 223
Herpetic, ... 223
Incubation of, ... 221
Indurations of, ... 222
Infection of, ... 221
Location of, ... 221
Mixed, ... 222
Number of, ... 223
Pain of, ... 223
Soft, ... 202
Treatment of, ... 226
Chancroids, ... 202
  Bubo of, ... 214
  Clinical History of, . . . 203
  Diphtheritic, ... 208
  Etiology of, ... 202
  Follicular, ... 208
  Gangrenous, ... 207
  Incubation of, ... 203
  Inoculation of, ... 203
  Location of, in Females, 206
  Of Anus, ... 206
  Phagedænic, ... 207
  Urethral, ... 206
  Treatment of, ... 208
  Abortive Treatment of, . 208
  Prophylactic Treatment of, 208
  Symptomatic Treatment of, 210
  Special Therapy for, . . 26–32
Chorea, Syphilitic, ... 283
Chordee, ... 34
  Treatment of, ... 40
Choroiditis, Syphilitic, . . . 253
  Disseminata, ... 253
Choroido-Retinitis, Syphi-
  litic, ... 254
  Treatment of, ... 255
Circumcision, ... 23
  Forceps, ... 23
Civiale's Meatotome, . . . 51
Colic, Renal, ... 137
Coma, Syphilitic, ... 284
Condylomata, ... 19, 64
  Special Therapy for, . 26–32

INDEX. 303

Conical Shaped Sounds, . . 52
Conjunctiva, Mucous Patches
   of, in Syphilis, ... 243
Conjunctivitis, Gonorrhœal, 77
   Etiology of, ... 77
   Clinical History of, . 78
   Treatment of, ... 82
   Special Therapy for, . . 83
   Syphilitic, ... 243
Cornea, Syphilis of, ... 243
   Gummy Infiltrations in, . 243
Cowperitis, ... 46, 87
   Etiology of, ... 87
   Clinical History of, . . 87
   Treatment of, . . . 46, 88
Cock's Operation for External
   Urethrotomy, ... 59
Cryptorchid, ... 156
Cutaneous Lesions of Sec-
   ondary Syphilis, . . 229
Cutaneous Lesions of Ter
   tiary Syphilis, . . . 270
Cyclitis, Syphilitic, ... 252
   Prognosis in, ... 252
   Treatment of, ... 252
Cystitis, ... 101
   Acute, ... 101
   Etiology of, ... 101
   Pathological Anatomy
      of, ... 102
   Clinical History of, . . 102
   Treatment of, ... 103
   Special Therapy for, 140-154
Cystitis, Chronic, ... 103
   Etiology of, ... 103
   Pathological Anatomy
      of, ... 103
   Clinical History of, . . 105
   Treatment of, ... 107
   Special Therapy for, 140-154
Cystitis, Gonorrhœal, . 46, 102
   Treatment of, ... 46
Cysts of the Testicle, . . . 172
   Treatment of, ... 172
   Special Therapy for, 179-184

D.

Dacryo-Adenitis, Syphilitic, 265
   Treatment of, ... 266
Dacryo-Cystitis, Syphilitic, 264
   Treatment of, ... 265
Diarrhœa in Syphilis, . . . 278
Diphtheritic Chancroid, . . 208
Divulsion of Stricture, . . 54
Divulsor, Thompson's . . . 54

E.

Ecthyma, of Secondary
   Syphilis, ... 233
   Treatment of, ... 235
   Tertiary, ... 270
   Treatment of. 272
Elephantiasis Scroti, ... 155
   Treatment of, ... 155
Endoscope, Otis', ... 35
   Perfected Otis, ... 35
Enuresis, ... 111
   Clinical History of, . . 111
   Treatment of, ... 111
   Special Therapy for, 140-154
English Catheter, ... 98
   Sounds, ... 53
Epididymitis, ... 165
   Etiology of, ... 165
   Pathological Anatomy
      of, ... 165
   Clinical History of, . . 166
   Treatment of, ... 167
   Special Therapy for, 179-184
Electrolysis for Resilient
   Strictures, ... 60
Electrolysis Sounds, New-
   man's, ... 59
Epilepsy, Syphilitic, . . . 283
Epithelioma of the Penis, . 21
   Etiology of, ... 21
   Clinical History of, . . 21
   Treatment of, ... 21
   Special Therapy for, . 26-32
Erythematous Syphilides, . 230
Erythematous Intertrigo of
   the Scrotum, ... 155

Extravasation of Urine, . . 61
External Urethrotomy, . . 56
Eyes, Venereal Diseases of,
       76, 243
 Amaurosis, ... 260
 Atrophy of Optic Nerve, . 259
 Choroiditis, ... 253
 Choroiditis, Disseminata, 253
 Choroido-Retinitis, . . . 254
  Treatment of, ... 255
 Conjunctiva, Syphilis of, 243
  Mucous Patches of, . . 243
  Gummy Infiltration of, 243
 Conjunctivitis, Gonor-
  rhœal, ... 77
 Cornea, Syphilis of, . . . 243
 Cyclitis, ... 252
  Prognosis in, ... 252
  Treatment of, ... 252
 Dacryo-Adenitis, ... 265
  Treatment of, ... 266
 Dacryo-cystitis, ... 264
  Treatment of, ... 265
 Gonorrhœal Conjunctivi-
  tis, ... 77
  Etiology of, ... 77
  Clinical History of, . . 78
  Prognosis of, ... 81
  Treatment of, ... 82
  Special Therapy for, . 83
 Gummy Scleritis, ... 247
 Hemianopsia, ... 260
  Treatment of, ... 260
 Inflammation of Lachry-
  mal Gland, ... 265
  Treatment of, ... 266
 Irido-Choroiditis, ... 252
  Treatment of, ... 253
 Iritis, Gonorrhœal, . . . 84
  Plastic Form — Clinical
   History of, ... 84
  Treatment of, ... 85
  Special Therapy for, . . 86
  Serous Form — Clinical
   History of, ... 85
  Treatment of, ... 87
  Special Therapy for, . . 87

Eyes (Continued).
 Iritis, Syphilitic, ... 248
  Etiology of, ... 248
  Clinical History of, . . 248
  Papular Form, ... 249
  Gummous Form, . . . 250
  Prognosis in, ... 250
  Treatment of, ... 250
 Keratitis Parenchymatosa, 243
  Etiology of, . . . 243
  Pathology of, ... 244
  Vascular Form,
   Clinical History of, . 244
  Prognosis in, ... 246
  Non-Vascular Form, . 246
  Treatment of, ... 246
 Kerato-Malacia, . . . 247
  Clinical History of, . . 247
  Prognosis in, ... 247
  Treatment of, ... 247
 Lachrymal Apparatus, . . 264
 Lids, Syphilis of, ... 262
  Gummy Infiltrations of, 263
  Tarsitis, ... 263
  Treatment of, ... 264
 Motor Nerves, Syphilis of, 267
  Fourth Nerve, ... 268
  Sixth Nerve, ... 268
  Third Nerve, ... 267
 Papillitis, ... 258
 Papillo-Retinitis, ... 258
 Periostitis of the Orbit, . 266
  Treatment of, ... 267
 Pre-Lachrymal Abscess, . 265
 Retinal Irritation, ... 256
 Retinitis, ... 256
 Retinitis, Central Recur-
  rent, ... 257
 Retinitis, Diffuse, ... 256
  Clinical History of, . . 257
  Prognosis in, ... 257
 Retrobulbar Neuritis, . . 259
 Syphilis of, ... 543

F.

Facial Paralysis, Syphilitic, 283
False Passages in Urethra, . 60

Treatment of, ... 60
Female, Gonorrhœa in, . . 62
Female, Stone in Bladder of, 130
Fever, Syphilitic, ... 228
    Character of, ... 229
    Treatment of, ... 229
Fever, Urethral or Urinary, 71
    Etiology of, ... 71
    Clinical History of, . . 71
    Treatment of, ... 72
Filiform Bougies, Banks', . 60
Finger, Syphilis of, ... 280
Follicular Chancroid, . . . 208
Folliculitis, Peri-Urethral, . 36
    Treatment of, ... 46
Forceps, Lithotomy, ... 124
French Sounds, ... 53
Fungus of the Testicle, . . 171
    Clinical History of, . . 171
    Treatment of, ... 171
    Special Therapy for, 179-184

G.

Gangrenous Chancroid, . . 207
Glands of Skene, ... 64
    Vulvo-vaginal, ... 62
Glans Penis, Stripping of, . 22
Gleet, ... 36
    Treatment of, ... 36
    Special Therapy for, . 64-70
Gonococcus of Neisser, . 33, 37
    Microscopical Examination of, ... 37
Gonorrhœa, ... 33
    Etiology of, ... 33
    Clinical History of, . . 33
    Treatment of, ... 36
    General Treatment of, . 38
    Special Therapy for, . 64-70
    Bastard, ... 36
    Etiology of, ... 36
    Clinical History of, . . 36
    Treatment of, ... 37
    General Treatment of, . 38
    Special Therapy for, . 64-70
    Chronic, ... 36
    Female, in the 62

Etiology of, ... 62
Clinical History of, . . 62
Treatment of, ... 63
Special Therapy for, . 64-70
Gonorrhœal Conjunctivitis, 77
    Etiology of, ... 77
    Clinical History of, . . 78
    Treatment of, ... 82
    Special Therapy for, . . 83
Gonorrhœal Iritis, ... 84
    Plastic Form, ... 84
    Treatment of, ... 85
    Special Therapy for, . . 86
    Serous Form, ... 85
    Treatment of, ... 87
    Special Therapy for, . . 87
Gonorrhœal Rheumatism, . 73
    Etiology of, ... 73
    Clinical History of, . . 73
    Treatment of, ... 74
    Special Therapy for, . 74-76
Gorget, Teale's, ... 57
Gouley's Operation in External Urethrotomy, . 58
Gravel, ... 135
    Clinical History of, . . 135
    Treatment of, ... 136
    Special Therapy for, 140-154
Gummata in Tertiary Syphilis, ... 272
    Of Bone, ... 280
        Treatment of, ... 280
    Of the Brain, ... 281
    Of Cartilage, ... 280
    Of the Larynx, ... 275
        Treatment of, ... 276
    Of the Liver, ... 279
        Treatment of, ... 279
    Of the Lungs, ... 277
        Treatment of, ... 277
    Of the Meninges, ... 281
    Of the Mucous Membranes, 273
        Treatment of, ... 274
    Of the Muscles, ... 280
    Of the Skin, ... 272
        Treatment of, ... 273
    Of the Spleen, ... 279

Of the Tongue, ... 274
    Treatment of, . . . 274
Gummy Scleritis, ... 247

H.

Hæmatocele, ... 162
    Etiology of, ... 162
    Acute, Clinical History of, 162
        Treatment of, ... 163
        Special Therapy for, 179–184
    Chronic, Clinical History
        of, ... 163
        Treatment of, ... 164
        Special Therapy for, 179–184
    Encysted, ... 165
        Treatment of, ... 165
        Special Therapy for, 179–184
    Of the Cord, ... 165
        Treatment of, ... 165
        Special Therapy for, 179–184
Hæmorrhage after Urethrotomy, ... 55
Hæmostat, Bates's Urethral, 55
Hair, Syphilis of, ... 236
Headache, Syphilitic, . . . 282
Helmuth's Supra-Pubic Operation for Removal of Stone, . . . 121
Hemianopsia in Syphilis, . 260
Hemiplegia, Syphilitic, . . 282
Hepatitis, Syphilitic, . . . 279
Hernia Testis, ... 171
    Clinical History of, . 171
    Treatment of, ... 171
    Special Therapy for, 179–184
Hereditary Syphilis, ... 286
    Treatment of, ... 287
    Special Therapy for, 295–300
Herpes Progenitalis, ... 18
    Etiology of, ... 19
    Treatment of, ... 19
    Preventive Treatment
        of, ... 19
    Special Therapy for, . 26–32
Hutchinson's Teeth, ... 287
Hydrocele, Acute, ... 156
    Treatment of, ... 156
    Special Therapy for,
        162, 179–184
Hydrocele, Chronic, ... 156
    Etiology of, ... 157
    Clinical History of, . . 157
    Surgical Treatment of, . 158
    Special Therapy for,
        162, 179–184
    Congenital, ... 160
        Treatment of, ... 161
        Special Therapy for,
        162, 179–184
Hydrocele of the Cord, . . 161
    Diffuse, ... 161
        Treatment of, ... 161
        Special Therapy for,
        162, 179–184
    Encysted, ... 161
        Treatment of, ... 162
        Special Therapy for,
        162, 179–184
Hypertrophy of the Prostate, 93
    Etiology of, ... 93
    Pathological Anatomy
        of, ... 93
    Clinical History of, . . 95
    Treatment of, ... 97
    Special Therapy for, 140–154
Hypertrophy of the Testicle, 155
Hypodermic Injections of
    Mercury, ... 293

I.

Impotence, ... 184
    False or Nervous, ... 187
        Etiology of, ... 187
        Clinical History of, . . 187
        Treatment of, ... 187
        Special Therapy for, 195–201
    True, ... 184
        Treatment of, ... 185
        Special Therapy for, 195–201
Incontinence of Urine, . . . 111
    Clinical History of, . . 111
    Treatment of, ... 111
    Special Therapy for, 140–154

Infiltration of Urine, Complicating Stricture from Rupture Behind It, . 61
Inflammatory Bubo, ... 212
Inflammatory Phimosis, . . 24
 Treatment of, ... 25
 Special Therapy for, . 26–32
Injections, Urethral, ... 42
 Technique of, ... 42
 For Deep Urethral, . . . 44
Insanity, Syphilitic, ... 284
Intertrigo of Scrotum, . . . 155
Intestines, Syphilis of, . . 277
Internal Urethrotomy, . . 54
Introduction of Sounds, . . 52
Irido-Choroiditis, Syphilitic, 252
Iritis, Gonorrhœal, ... 84
 Plastic Form, ... 84
 Treatment of, ... 85
 Serous Form, ... 85
 Treatment of, ... 87
Iritis, Syphilitic, ... 248
Irritability of the Bladder, . 109
 Etiology of, ... 109
 Clinical History of, . . 109
 Treatment of, ... 110
 Special Therapy for, 140-154
Irritable Testicle, ... 175
 Etiology of, ... 175
 Clinical History of, . . 175
 Treatment of, ... 175
 Special Therapy for, 179-184
Irritation of the Neck of the Bladder in Gonnorhœa, ... 40, 102
 Treatment of, ... 40

K.

Keratitis Parenchymatosa, Syphilitic, ... 243
Kerato-Malacia, Syphilitic, 247
 Clinical History of, . . 247
 Prognosis in, ... 247
 Treatment of, ... 247
Keyes' Tonic Treatment in Syphilis, ... 290

Keyes - Ultzmann's Deep Urethral Syringe, . . 44
Keyes' Varicocele Needle, . . 177
Kidney, Syphilis of, ... 279
 Congestion of, ... 279
 Treatment, ... 280
 Nephritis, ... 281
 Treatment of, ... 247
Kidney, Abscess of Pelvis of, 134
Kiefer's Two-way Tube, . . 40
Knife, Blunt Meatotomy, . 50
 Lithotomy, ... 123
 Probe-pointed, ... 123

L.

Lachrymal Apparatus, Syphilis of, ... 264
Larynx, Syphilis of, ... 275
 Erythema of, ... 275
 Superficial Ulcers of, . . 275
 Tertiary Symptoms of, . . 275
 Ulcers, Deep, of, ... 275
 Prognosis in, ... 276
 Treatment of, ... 276
Lids, Syphilis of, ... 262
Litholapaxy, ... 127
Lithotrite, Bigelow's, . . . 127
Lithotomy Forceps, ... 124
 Knife, ... 123
 Median, ... 124
 Staff, ... 122
 Supra-Pubic, ... 125
Liver, Syphilis of, ... 279
 Diffuse Parenchymatous Hyperplasia of, . . . 279
 Gummata of, ... 279
 Clinical History of, . . 279
 Treatment of, ... 279
Lungs, Syphilis of, ... 276
 Fibrinous Interstitial Pneumonia, ... 277
 Gummata of, ... 277
 White Hepatization of, . 276
 Treatment of, ... 277
Lymphangitis, in Gonorrhœa, ... 35

Treatment of, ... 46
Lymphatics in Syphilis, . . 224

M.

Marcy's Double Current
    Catheter, ... 107
Marriage, Syphilis and, . . 285
Masturbation, ... 189
    Clinical History of, . . 190
    Treatment of, ... 190
    Special Therapy for, 195-201
Meatus Urinarius, Stricture
    of, ... 50
Meatotomy, ... 50
  With Blunt-Pointed Knife, 50
  With Civiale's Meatotome, 51
Mercier's Catheter, ... 98
Mercury in Syphilis, . . . 289
  Baehr Advises, ... 290
  Hahnemann Advises, . . 289
  Jahr Advises, ... 290
  Jousset Advises, ... 290
  Keyes Advises, ... 290
  Yeldham Advises, . . . 290
  Hypodermics of, . . . 293
  Inunctions of, ... 291
  Fumigation with, . . . 292
Miscarriage, due to Syphilis, ... 285
Misemissions, ... 189
Monorchids, ... 156
Motor Nerves of the Eye, 267
  Syphilis of, ... 267
  Fourth Nerve, ... 268
  Sixth Nerve, ... 268
  Third Nerve, ... 267
Mucous Membrane, Lesions
  of, in Second Stage of
  Syphilis, ... 239
Mucous Patches, ... 240
  Prognosis in, ... 241
  Treatment of, ... 241
  Scaly Patches, ... 241
  Treament of, ... 241
Mucous Membranes in Tertiary Stage of Syphilis, ... 273

Mucous Patches, ... 273
Gummatous Ulcerations, . . 273
  Treatment of, ... 274
Muscles, Syphilis of, . . . 280
  Treatment of, ... 281
Gummatous Infiltration
  of, ... 280
  Treatment of, ... 281
Syphilitic Rheumatism, . 280
  Treatment of, ... 281

N.

Nails, Syphilis of, ... 238
  Treatment of, ... 239
Needle, Keyes' Varicocele, . 177
Neisser's Gonococcus, . . 33, 37
Nervous System, Syphilis of, 281
  Aphasia, Syphilitic, . . 283
  Cephalalgia, Syphilitic, 282
  Chorea, Syphilitic, . . 283
  Coma, Syphilitic, . . . 284
  Epilepsy, Syphilitic, . . 283
  Facial Paralysis, Syphilitic, ... 283
  Hemiplegia, Syphilitic 282
  Insanity, Syphilitic, . . 284
  Paraplegia, Syphilitic, . 284
Neuralgia of the Bladder, . 109
  Etiology of, ... 109
  Clinical History of, . . 109
  Treatment of, ... 110
  Special Therapy for, 140-154
Neuralgia of the Testes, . . 175
  Etiology of, ... 175
  Clinical History of, . . 175
  Treatment of, ... 175
  Special Therapy for, 179-184
Newman's Electrolysis
  Sounds, ... 60
Nietze's Cystoscope, . . . 104
Nymphomania, ... 191
  Treatment of, ... 191
  Special Therapy for, 195-201

O.

Onanism, ... 189
  Clinical History of, . . 190

INDEX.

Treatment of, ... 190
    Special Therapy for, 195-201
Onychia, Syphylitic, . . . 238
    Treatment of, ... 239
Orchitis, ... 169
    Acute, ... 170
        Etiology of, ... 170
        Clinical History of, . . 170
        Treatment of, ... 170
        Special Therapy for, 179-184
    Chronic, ... 170
        Etiology of, ... 170
        Clinical History of, . . 170
        Treatment of, ... 171
        Special Therapy for, 179-184
    Syphilitic, ... 171
        Etiology of, ... 171
        Clinical History of, . . 171
        Treatment of, ... 171
        Special Therapy for, 179-184
Otis' Endoscope, ... 35
    Perfected, ... 35
    Scale, Urethral, ... 50
    Urethrometer, ... 44
    Urethrotome, ... 54

P.

Papillitis, Syphilitic, . . . 258
Papular Syphilides, . . . 230
Papulo-Retinitis, Syphilitic, 258
Paraphimosis, ... 25
    Etiology of, ... 25
    Clinical History of, . . 25
    Treatment of, ... 25
    Special Therapy for, . 26-32
Paraplegia, Syphilitic, . . 284
Paronychia, Syphilitic, . . 238
    Treatment of, ... 239
Pediculi Pubis, ... 154
    Treatment of, ... 154
Penis, Epithelioma of, . . 21
    Etiology of, ... 21
    Clinical History of, . . 21
    Treatment of, ... 21
    Special Therapy for, . 26-32
Perinæal Section in External
    Urethrotomy, ... 59

Phagedænic Chancroid, . . 207
Phimosis, ... 21
    Etiology of, ... 21
    Clinical History of, . . 21
    Treatment of, ... 22
    Forceps, ... 23
    Inflammatory, ... 24
    Treatment of, ... 25
    Special Therapy for, . 26-32
Phtheriasis Pubis, ... 154
    Treatment of, ... 154
Pigmentary Syphilides, . . 233
Pollutions, ... 192
    Diurnal, ... 193
    Treatment of, ... 193
    Special Therapy for, 195-201
    Nocturnal, ... 192
    Treatment of, ... 193
    Special Therapy for, 195-201
Posthitis, ... 17
    Etiology of, ... 17
    Clinical History of, . . 17
    Prognosis in, ... 18
    Treatment of, ... 18
    Special Therapy for, . 26-32
Pregnancy, Syphilis and . . 285
Prepuce, Varices of, ... 20
    Treatment of, ... 20
Preputial Calculi, ... 20
    Treatment, ... 21
Priapism, ... 191
    Clinical History of, . . 192
    Treatment of, ... 192
    Special Therapy for, 195-201
Prostatitis, Acute, ... 88
    Etiology of, ... 88
    Pathological Anatomy
        of, ... 88
    Clinical History of, . . 88
    Treatment of, ... 89
    Special Therapy for, 140-154
    Chronic or Follicular, . . 90
    Etiology of, ... 90
    Pathological Anatomy
        of, ... 90
    Clinical History of, . . 90

Treatment of, ... 90
Special Therapy for, 140-154
Tubercular, ... 92
Prostate, Hypertrophy of, . 93
   Etiology of, ... 93
   Pathological Anatomy
     of, ... 93
   Clinical History of, . . 95
   Treatment of, ... 97
   Special Therapy for, 140-154
Psychrophor, ... 93
Prurigo Genitalia, ... 155
   Treatment of, ... 155
Pustular Syphilides, ... 232
   Acne, ... 233
   General Superficial, . . . 232
   Ecthyma, Superficial, . . 233
Pustules of Tertiary Stage,
   of Syphilis, ... 271
Pyelitis, ... 132
   Acute, ... 132
   Chronic, ... 132
   Calculous, ... 132
   Tubercular, ... 132
   Clinical History of, . . . 133
     Acute, ... 133
     Chronic, ... 134
   Pathological Anatomy
     of, ... 132
   Treatment of, ... 134
   Special Therapy for, 140-154

R.

Rectum, Syphilis of, . . . 278
   Stricture of, ... 278
   Clinical History of, . . 278
   Treatment of, ... 278
Renal Calculi, ... 137
Renal Colic, ... 137
   Clinical History of, . . 137
   Treatment of, ... 138
   Special Therapy for, 140-154
Resilient Stricture of the
   Urethra, ... 60
   Treatment of, ... 60
Retention of Urine, ... 113
   Clinical History of, . . 113
   Treatment of, ... 114

Special Therapy for, 140-154
Retinitis, Syphilitic. 256
Retrobulbar Neuritis, Syph-
   ilitic, ... 259
Retinal Irritation, Syphilitic, 256
Retinitis, Diffuse Syphilitic, 256
   Clinical History of, . . 257
   Prognosis in, ... 257
Rheumatism, Gonorrhœal, . 73
   Etiology of, ... 73
   Clinical History of, . . 73
   Treatment of, ... 74
   Special Therapy for, . 74-76
   Syphilitic, ... 280
   Treatment of, ... 281
Ricord's Circumcision For-
   ceps, ... 23
Roseola, Syphilitic, ... 230
Rubber Syringe, Universal, 42
Rupia, Syphilitic, ... 270

S.

Salivation from Mercury, . 242
   Treatment of, ... 242
Satyriasis, ... 191
   Treatment of, ... 191
   Special Therapy for, 195-201
Self-Abuse, ... 189
Scaly Patches of Mucous
   Membrane in Syphi-
   lis, ... 241
Scrotum, Cutaneous Dis-
   eases of, ... 155
   Elephantiasis of, ... 155
   Treatment of, ... 155
   Erythematous Intertrigo, 155
   Treatment of, ... 155
   Prurigo of, ... 155
   Treatment of, ... 155
Secondary Stage of Syphlis, 227
Silver Catheter with Long
   Curve, ... 98
Simple Bubo, ... 212
Skene's Glands, ... 64
   Ducts, ... 64
Skene's Apparatus to Douche
   the Bladder, ... 107

Sounds, Conical-Shaped, . . 52
    English, ... 53
    French, ... 53
    Introduction of, ... 52–53
    Weisse's, ... 51
Spermatorrhœa, ... 192
    Etiology of, ... 193
    Clinical History of, . . 194
    Treatment of, ... 195
    Special Therapy for, 195-201
Spleen, Syphilis of, ... 279
Squamous Syphilides, . . . 234
Sterility, ... 188
    Treatment of, ... 188
    Special Therapy for, 195-201
Staff, Lithotomy, ... 122
    Symes's, ... 58
Stomach, Syphilis of, . . . 277
Stone in Bladder, ... 115
    Etiology of, ... 116
    Clinical History of, . . 116
    Non-operative Treat-
      ment of, ... 120
    Operative Treatment of, 121
Stone in Bladder of Female, 130
    Treatment of, ... 131
Stricture, ... 46
    Annular, ... 48
    Divulsion of, ... 54
    Electrolysis in, ... 60
    Irregular, ... 48
    Internal Urethrotomy in, . 54
    Linear, ... 48
    Meatus of, ... 50
      Operation for, ... 50
    Resilient, ... 60
    Organic, ... 48
    Spasmodic, ... 46
    Etiology of, ... 46
    Clinical History of, . . 47
    Treatment of, ... 47
    Special Therapy for, . 64-70
Strangury, ... 114
    Treatment of, ... 114
Stripping of Glans Penis, . . 22
Syphilides, ... 229

Bulbous, ... 234
Characteristics of, ... 229
Color of, ... 229
Erythematous, ... 230
    Treatment of, ... 235
Papular, ... 230
    Small Pointed, ... 231
    Large Pointed, ... 231
    Small Flat, ... 231
    Large Flat, ... 231
    Palms of Hands of, . . 232
    Treatment of, ... 235
Pigmentary, ... 233
Pustular, ... 232
    Acne, ... 233
    Ecthyma, Superficial, . 233
    General Superficial, . . 232
    Treatment of, ... 235
Roseola, ... 230
    Treatment of, ... 235
Squamous, ... 234
    Treatment of, ... 235
Tubercular, ... 234
    Circular Groups, . . . 234
    General, ... 234
    Treatment of, ... 235
Vesicular, ... 234
    Treatment of, . . . 235
Syphilis, ... 219
    Etiology of, ... 220
    Clinical History of, . . 221
    Diagnosis from Chan-
      croid, ... 224
    Primary Stage of, ... 221
    Treatment of, ... 226
    Secondary Stage of, . . 227
    Treatment of,
        235, 236, 239, 241
    Tertiary Stage of, ... 269
      Treatment of, ... 272
    General Treatment of, . 288
    Special Therapy for, 295-300
    Baths in, ... 288
Syphilis, ... 219
    Alopecia of, ... 236
    Treatment of, ... 236
    Abortion Due to, ... 285

Syphilis (Continued).
  Cutaneous Lesions in, . . 229
  Diarrhœa of, ... 278
  Duration of, ... 226
  Fever of, ... 228
    Treatment of, ... 229
  Glandular Enlargement
    in, ... 228
  Hot Springs in, ... 289
  Incubation of, ... 221
  Secondary Stage of, . . . 227
  Infantile, ... 285
  Influence of age in, . . . 219
    Climate in, ... 219
    Gout in, ... 219
    Scrofula in, ... 219
  Inherited, ... 286
    Appearance of, ... 286
    Countenance in, ... 287
    Treatment of, ... 287
  Inoculation of, . . . 220
  Mucous Membrane in Second Stage of, ... 239
  Mucous Patches, ... 240
    Scaly Patches, ... 241
    Prognosis in, ... 241
    Treatment of, . . . 241
  Mucous Patches in Tertiary Stage. . . . 273
    Deep Ulcerations, . . . 273
    Gummatous Ulceration, 273
    Treatment of, ... 274
  Of the Anus, ... 278
    Treatment of, . . 278
  Of the Brain, ... 281
    Treatment of, . . . 285, 289
  Of Bones, ... 280
    Treatment of, ... 280
  Of the Eye, ... 243
    Choroiditis, ... 253
    Choroiditis Disseminata, 253
    Choroido-Retinitis, . . 254
    Treatment of, ... 255
    Conjunctiva, ... 243
    Mucous Patches of, . . 243
    Gummy Infiltrations of, 243
    Cornea, Keratitis Parenchymatosa, ... 243

Syphilis (Continued).
  Etiology of, ... 243
  Pathology of, ... 244
  Clinical History of Vascular Forms, . 244
  Prognosis in, ... 246
  Non-Vascular Form, . 246
  Treatment of, ... 246
  Cyclitis, ... 252
    Prognosis in, . . . 252
    Treatment of, ... 252
  Gummy Infiltration of Conjunctiva, . . 243
  Gummy Scleritis, . . . 247
  Irido-Choroiditis, . . . 252
  Iritis, ... 248
    Etiology of, . . 248
    Clinical History of, . 248
    Papular Form of, . . 249
    Prognosis in, ... 250
    Treatment of, ... 250
  Kerato-Malacia, ... 247
    Clinical History of, . 247
    Prognosis in, ... 247
    Treatment of, ... 247
  Motor Nerves, ... 267
    Fourth Nerve, . . . 268
    Sixth Nerve, . . . 268
    Third Nerve, or Motor Oculi, ... 268
  Papillitis and Papillo-Retinitis, ... 258
  Periostitis of the Orbit, 266
    Treatment of, ... 267
  Retinitis, ... 256
  Retinal Irritation, . . . 256
  Retinitis, Central Recurrent, ... 257
  Diffuse, ... 256
    Clinical History of, . 257
    Prognosis in, ... 257
    Treatment of, ... 257
  Of the Fingers, ... 280
    Treatment of, ... 281
  Of the Intestines, . . . 277
    Treatment of, ... 278
  Of the Kidney, ... 279
    Congestion of, . . . 279

Treatment of, ... 280
Nephritis in, ... 280
Treatment of, ... 280
Of the Larynx, ... 275
Erythema of, ... 275
Superficial Ulcers of, . 275
Tertiary Symptoms of, 275
Ulcers of, ... 275
Prognosis in, ... 276
Treatment of, ... 276
Of the Liver, ... 279
  Diffuse Parenchymatous
    Hyperplasia of, . . . 279
Gummata of, ... 279
Clinical History of, . . 279
Treatment of, ... 279
Of the Lungs, ... 276
  Fibrous Interstitial Pneu-
    monia in, ... 277
Gummata of, ... 277
White Hepatization in, 276
Treatment of, ... 277
Of the Muscles, ... 280
Rheumatism of, . . . 280
Treatment of, ... 281
Gummata of, ... 280
Treatment of, ... 281
Of Mucous Membranes,
                239, 273
Mucous Patches, . 239, 273
Scaly Patches, ... 240
Prognosis in, ... 241
Treatment of, . . 241, 274
Ulceration, Gummatous, 273
Treatment of, ... 274
Of the Nails, ... 238
Treatment of, ... 239
Of the Nervous System, . 281
Aphasia in, ... 283
Cephalalgia in, ... 282
Chorea in, ... 283
Coma in, ... 284
Epilepsy in, ... 283
Facial Paralysis in, . . 283
Hemiplegia in, ... 282
Insanity in, ... 284
Paraplegia in, ... 284

Of the Orpital Nerves, . . 267
Of the Rectum, ... 278
Stricture of, ... 278
Clinical History of, . . 278
Treatment of, ... 287
Of the Tendons, ... 280
Of the Tongue, ... 274
Gummata of, . . . 274
Treatment of, ... 274
Paronychia, ... 238
Treatment of, ... 239
Primary Stage, ... 221
Treatment of, ... 226
Second Inoculation of, . 223
Secondary Stage of, . . 227
Treatment of, 235, 236, 241
Secretions, Infectious Na-
  ture of, ... 220
Tertiary Stage, ... 269
Cutaneous Diseases of, . 270
Appearance of, ... 270
Ecthyma in, ... 270
Treatment of, . . . 272
Gummatous Deposits in, 272
Of the Skin in, ... 272
Treatment of, ... 272
Pustules in, ... 271
Treatment of, ... 272
Rupia in, ... 270
Treatment of, ... 272
Ulceration in, ... 271
Superficial, of, . . . 271
Deep, of, ... 271
Treatment of, ... 272

T.

Taylor's Deep Urethral
  Syringe, ... 44
Teale's Gorget, ... 57
Tendons, Syphilis of, . . . 280
Testicle, Absence of, . . . 156
Atrophy of, ... 156
Cancer of, ... 172
Treatment of, . . . 173
Special Therapy for, 179-184
Cysts of, ... 172
Treatment of, ... 172

Special Therapy for, 179-184
Encysted Hydrocele of, . . 161
Hernia of, ... 171
 Clinical History of, . . 171
 Treatment of, ... 171
 Special Therapy for, 179-184
Hypertrophy of, ... 155
Inflammation of, ... 169
Irritability of, ... 175
 Etiology of, ... 175
 Clinical History of, . . 175
 Treatment of, . . 175
 Special Therapy for, 179-184
Neuralgia of, ... 175
 Etiology of, ... 175
 Clinical History of, . . 175
 Treatment of, ... 175
 Special Therapy for, 179-184
Removal of, ... 174
 Clinical History of, . . 171
 Treatment of, ... 171
 Special Therapy for, 179-184
Syphilis of, ... 171
Strapping of, ... 169
Tubercular, ... 173
 False, ... 173
 Etiology of, ... 173
 Clinical History of, . . 173
 Treatment of, ... 173
 Special Therapy for, 179-184
 True, ... 173
 Pathological Anatomy
  of, ... 173
 Clinical History of, . . 174
 Treatment of, ... 174
 Special Therapy for, 179-184
Thermo-Galvanic Treatment
 of Hypertrophy of the
 Prostate, ... 100
Thompson's Divulsor . . . 54
Thompson's Stone Searcher, 97
Tobin's Operation for Hypertrophy of the Prostate. 100
Tongue, Gummata of, . . . 274
 Treatment of, ... 274
Tunneled Catheter, ... 57

Trendelenburg's Position, . . 125
Tubercular Syphilides, . . 234
 Circular Groups, ... 234
 General, ... 234

U.

Ulcers, Syphilitic, of Skin, . 271
 Deep, ... 271
 Superficial, ... 271
 Treatment of, ... 272
Universal Soft-Rubber Syringe, ... 42
Urethra, False Passages of, 60
 Treatment of, ... 61
Urethra, Stricture of, . . . 46
 Impassable, ... 71
Urethral Discharges, General Treatment of, . . 38
Urethral Fever, ... 53, 71
 Etiology of, ... 71
 Clinical History of, . . . 71
 Treatment of, ... 72
Urethral Hæmostat, Bates', 55
Urethral Injections, Technique of, ... 42
Urethral Vegetations, . . . 36
Urethritis, ... 37
 Etiology of, ... 37
 Clinical History of, . . . 37
 Treatment of, ... 38
 General, Treatment of, . . 38
 Special Therapy for, . . 64-70
Urethrococcus, ... 37
 Microscopical Examination of, ... 37
Urethrometer, Otis', ... 44
Urethroscope, Otis', ... 35
Urethroscope, Perfected, . . 35
Urethrotome, Otis', ... 54
Urinary Fever, ... 71

V.

Varices of the Prepuce, . . 20
 Treatment of, ... 21
 Special Therapy for, . 26-32
Varicocele, ... 176
 Etiology of, ... 176

Clinical History of, . . 176
Treatment of, ... 177
Special Therapy for,
    178, 179–184
Varicocele Needle, Keyes', . 177
Vegetations, ... 19
    Etiology of, ... 19
    Clinical History of, . . 19
    Treatment of, ... 19
    Special Therapy for, . 26–32
    Of the Urethra, ... 36
Venereal Warts, ... 19
    Treatment of, ... 19
    Special Therapy for, . 26–32
Vesical Calculus, ... 115
    Etiology of, ... 116
    Clinical History of, . . 116
    Non-operative Treatment
        of, ... 120
Operative Treatment for, 121
    In the Female, ... 130
    Treatment of, ... 131
Vesical Tenesmus, ... 114
    Treatment of, ... 114
    Special Therapy for, 140-154
Virulent Bubo, ... 214

W.

Warts, Venereal, ... 19
    Etiology of, ... 19
    Clinical History of, . 19
    Treatment of, ... 19
    Special Therapy for, . 26–32
Weisse's Sounds, ... 51
Wheelhouse's External Urethrotomy, ... 59
White's Operation for Castration in Hypertrophy of the Prostate, . 101

www.ingramcontent.com/pod-product-compliance
Lightning Source LLC
Chambersburg PA
CBHW031905220426
43663CB00006B/768